Geriatric Education

Geriatric Education

edited by
KNIGHT STEEL, M.D.

Chief, Geriatrics Section
Evans Memorial Department of Clinical
Research and Department of Medicine
University Hospital
Boston University Medical Center
and
Chief, Section of Teachers of Geriatric Medicine
American Geriatrics Society

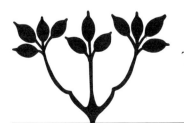

THE COLLAMORE PRESS
D.C. Heath and Company
Lexington, Massachusetts
Toronto

Published simultaneously in Canada and the United Kingdom

Printed in the United States of America

International Standard Book Number: 0–669–03809–1

Library of Congress Catalog Card Number: 80–832

Library of Congress Cataloging in Publication Data
Main entry under title:

Geriatric education

   "The majority of papers included . . . were originally
given at the Third Inter-University Conference on
Geriatric Medicine of the American Geriatrics Society."
   Includes index.
   1. Geriatrics–Study and teaching–Congresses.
I. Steel, Knight. II. Inter-University Conference on
Geriatric Medicine, 3d, Chicago, 1980. [DNLM:
1. Geriatrics–Education, WT 18 G369]
RC952.5.G43   618.97'0071   80–832
ISBN 0–669–03809–1

To my wife, Elizabeth, and my children, Ashley and Gillian—
inhabitants of Mole End

Contents

Foreword

One could assert that the striking prolongation of the average human lifespan during the twentieth century deserves to be listed among the major events of our time, together with such innovations as air travel, mass communication, atomic energy, and exploration of space. Rather abruptly, we have had to recognize that we are members of a population containing tens of millions of people who are beyond the age of childrearing or economic productivity.

This situation poses cultural, social, and economic problems, which cannot be coped with solely by the medical profession; nevertheless, medicine is drawn into it, perhaps to a greater extent than any other profession. We are going to be called on increasingly to do what we can for chronic progressive disabilities of elderly patients. To do that well, we need to understand the realities of their position in our youth-oriented society. As things stand now, there is reason to wonder whether our grandchildren will be proud of us, as they look back at the way we have provided for this first impact of a large community of old people. The truth is, we simply cannot walk away from it, ignoring conditions that cause the elderly to be more or less forgotten and hidden away.

Assuredly, the practice of medicine already involves geriatrics but that is largely in management of acute illness. Outside the hospital, we pay too little attention to the circumstances in which the elderly have to exist or to the kind of help available to them. Elderly people are subject not only to acute illnesses but also to multiple, chronic disabilities; and that at a time when they are also having to contend with personal losses, as well as social, psychological, and economic handicaps.

In the United States, the system of health-care delivery is geared to acute illness, with emphasis on technological procedures for diagnosis and treatment, but that may not be the major requirement for care of the geriatric population. We should be alerting the public and politicians that many things could be done to promote the welfare and functional independence of the elderly.

One of the obvious targets of our attention should be long-term-care institutions. These too often are just domiciles where elderly dependent people are kept out of sight. The atmosphere may be of defeat, the food monotonous and tasteless, and the attendants impatient and ill-trained.

Unfortunately, our welfare and health services are fragmented and uncoordinated, with payment favoring a system that rewards acute hospital care. If we could improve the organization of our medical and welfare services, the result would be a better quality of life for our older citizens at less cost to taxpayers. We owe it to our patients and fellow citizens, indeed eventually to ourselves, to try to improve the quality of life of the aged and, at the same time, lessen the cost of their care.

This volume, containing contributions presented at the Third Inter-University Conference on Geriatric Education, under the auspices of the American Geriatrics Society, presents an interesting cross-section of the ways in which a growing band of dedicated workers is testing methods to improve the welfare of our older citizens.

Paul B. Beeson

Preface

During the late 1970s, geriatric medicine rather suddenly was received with a surge of enthusiasm. The lay press and even traditional medical journals published articles about the health-care needs of the elderly. Conferences directed at geriatric medicine and the diseases of old age, predominantly at the level of postgraduate medical education, abounded. The federal government offered funds for the development of programs in geriatrics at the undergraduate and graduate levels of medical education.

What has become apparent to the increasing numbers of persons interested in geriatric medicine is the need to institutionalize programs that were subsidized by granting agencies initially for only a limited time. In order for a teaching effort to endure beyond the life of a grant or the impetus engendered by the still-small number of faculty, geriatrics must find its place within the structure of academic medicine. Given both the demands for time in the curriculum by more-established units and subunits and the limited resources available to all, it is clear that geriatric medicine faces significant problems in the 1980s.

Solutions to these difficulties will be designed with greater ease and implemented with greater success when the problems are delineated more clearly. Whether geriatrics eventually becomes a unique specialty, with or without a certifying examination, or whether it should is not at issue here. Rather, the authors of this book address four concerns, which are of special importance to the development of credibility for geriatrics within academic medicine.

Today, most of the physicians who staff hospitals and long-term-care facilities, in addition to those who practice or teach in other settings, received their training under the American system of medical education and university-affiliated hospitals. The need to improve the quality of care for the elderly by implementing changes in the American program of medical education has been raised repeatedly by the American Geriatrics Society as well as by other professional and lay organizations. The report of the Committee on Geriatric Medicine of the Institute of Medicine, the National Academy of Sciences [1], detailed some of the profound defects in the way geriatric medicine has been taught within medical schools and postgraduate training programs and made recommendations for change. Whether or not their suggestions or those of others are accepted by all concerned, it is in the academic setting that the resources of space, faculty, and money must be garnered if a change in the product of medical education is to take place, which in turn is necessary for improving the care of the older generation.

Furthermore, since some increased knowledge about aging and the needs of and management of the elderly population is essential for almost all physicians who will practice medicine in the next 50 years, the need for a change in educational programs is not limited to that necessary for the training of a small contingent of medical students. Almost 33 percent of the 1 million or so acute-care hospital beds and about 90 percent of the 1.2 million chronic-care beds in the United States are presently occupied by those 65 years of age and over, although that segment of the population comprises only about 11 percent of the whole. Not only are the aged now utilizing a markedly disproportionate percentage of our health-care system but the present-day trend of yet-increasing numbers of older persons (especially a relative increase in the numbers of frail elderly) will continue in all likelihood. Thus, only a few physicians, such as obstetricians who opt not to include gynecology in their work and some pediatricians, may be truly unaffected by the demographics of our nation.

Before considering the four issues that seem especially critical to the establishment of geriatric medicine, a sense of the recent history of its development is required. Therefore, the first section of the book is an overview adapted from the State-of-the-Art Lecture given at the Annual Meeting of the American College of Physicians in New Orleans in April 1980.

The second section, edited by T. Franklin Williams, M.D., addresses the kinds of facilities necessary for the teaching and practice of geriatric medicine. It must be remembered that little interest would likely be expressed by any of the classic subdivisions of academic medicine for events beyond the doors of the acute-care hospital. These traditional subunits have been based at acute tertiary-care hospitals not only because technological aspects of treatment and research require it but for other reasons as well. The need for conservation of the physician's time, reimbursement and financial considerations, and easy access to colleagues for collaboration in therapeutic and investigative procedures have all played a role in the development of the acute hospital as central to academic medicine.

Regretably, this model is not wholly appropriate for the practice of geriatric medicine. It can be said that no doctor would be willing to be called a geriatrician without an association with a long-term-care institution and, perhaps, a home-care program as well. Clearly this is not the case for most other academicians. Although departments of family practice have instituted some exceptions to this general policy, medical schools as a whole remain committed to the centrality of the acute-care hospital to the exclusion of other health-care settings. Thus, although rotations for house staff and students beyond the doors of the acute hospital are somewhat more prevalent, such experiences still are not commonplace and are rare for departments of medicine.

The experience of geriatrics in the United Kingdom is relevant to a discussion of settings for in that country it has been customary to saddle departments of geriatric medicine with the most antiquated buildings. This surely must have some effect on the teaching of the subject. Also with regard to clinical settings, although it is impossible to design a geriatric unit solely at an acute hospital, the acute-care setting as a resource for geriatric medicine requires special consideration, for it is there that so much of the training will surely take place.

The third section, edited by Gerald Gehringer, M.D., is concerned with the overlap between units of geriatric medicine and "primary-care medicine," be they departments of family practice or divisions of general medicine within a department of medicine. Unquestionably there are some potential problems in this area, since geriatric units and primary-care units may be vying for the same patients and for the fiscal stability that accompanies large patient-care units. It is not the intent of this book to consider whether programs in geriatric medicine should be located within departments of family practice or internal medicine. Nor should the importance of other departments within the medical school, especially departments of psychiatry, rehabilitation medicine, and neurology be slighted. However, I contend that relationships between units of primary-care medicine and geriatric medicine must be established within the academic setting if the best care for the elderly is to be made possible.

Then there is the problem of research. Unlike organ-system specialties, geriatric medicine has no specific area or turf within the body proper. Rather, in the future, researchers in geriatric medicine will be required to draw upon the skills and capabilities of subspecialists. Thus, it is envisioned that cardiologists interested in geriatric medicine, neurologists interested in geriatric medicine, and so on will adapt their special capabilities to the diseases prevalent in the aged.

By traditional standards, the elderly patient can be a poor subject for clinical investigation because the older person is not a "pure" model of disease. Multiple pathological entities as well as social factors can confound attempts to investigate a single disease state. Additionally, because of age and the presence of concomitant illness, the elderly person may be a high-risk subject for any invasive procedure used on an experimental basis. Nonetheless, research is essential if geriatric medicine is to produce new thoughts and knowledge and be accepted within academic medicine. Therefore, the fourth section is devoted to the critical role of research in the development of academic programs in geriatric medicine. Edited by John W. Rowe, M.D., this section demonstrates clearly the need for and the capability of carrying out research in six areas critical to the establishment of geriatric medicine. Included are chapters about geriatric problems where an alliance is achieved with the more traditional specialties of cardiology, neurology, metabolism, clinical pharmacology, and infectious disease. In addition, there is a chapter directed to aspects of health-care research and its important place in the future of geriatrics.

The fifth section addresses the very difficult matter of communication between departments. Classical units within a department of medicine or indeed most other departments are often rather well defined. If one wanted to establish a division of hematology, for example, I would contend that the requirements listed by a half a dozen people, knowledgeable and capable of establishing such a unit, would not be substantially different from one another.[1] Thus, at any of fifty major university hospitals in the country, the hematology division would have inpatient rights or perhaps a ward, one or two hematology clinics, an area for bench research, and a faculty of 3 to 10 persons with interests in red cells, white cells, platelets, and clotting. There would be physicians at the level of fellows who would respond to requests for consultation throughout the hospital and who would work in laboratories during a second year of training.

Persons in this division would relate rather tangentially and only where needed to other units within the department of medicine, except perhaps for a unique relationship with oncology. There would be few, if any, lines of communication with other departments in the medical school, such as neurology or psychiatry. This model has been exceptionally successful for the classic subdivisions within a department of medicine.

More important, schools of medicine have had little to do with other schools within the university. For example, there are occasional, almost random, collegial efforts with schools of nursing, but the number of collaborative efforts by physicians with nurses, not to mention social workers, occupational therapists, physical therapists, and even doctorate-level persons other than those in the basic sciences, are rare indeed.

Therefore, this section, edited by Stanley Brody, M.S.W., J.D., addresses the need for communication between medical schools and other health-related schools. Geriatric medicine has a unique requirement in this regard. How such relationships will be established is critical to the development of geriatric medicine itself. Will nurses have appointments in departments of medicine? Will doctors have appointments in schools of social work? Let me state emphatically that medical students will not be transformed into social workers as some might envision the aim of geriatrics, but it is equally inappropriate for medical students and physicians to be so lacking in knowledge of social welfare that patient care is not only fragmented (to use the catchword) but just plain poor.

A few specific examples of nursing roles are included elsewhere, but the chapters in this section are especially relevant to relationships between nursing schools and medical schools. New roles for the nursing profession are being established including responsibilities in large coronary care units, pediatric practices with one or more nurse practitioners, or dialysis units. The substantial role of the nurse in geriatric care has not always been recognized. Although the commitment of nursing professionals is not likely to decrease, better coordination of efforts between physicians and nurses, especially in geriatric medicine, seems advisable. This will require a new rapprochement between schools of medicine and nursing.

This book is limited in scope and reflective of a wide array of opinion. It is apparent that these four major issues—the selection of appropriate clinical sites for teaching, the special relationship between geriatric medicine and primary care, the development of a research base for geriatric medicine, and communication within the school of medicine and beyond—are among the most important and critical problems facing geriatric medicine at this time. Great effort should be directed to them if geriatric medicine is to gain substance in academia.

The majority of chapters in this book were originally given as papers at the Third Inter-University Conference on Geriatric Medicine of the American Geriatrics Society. The Conference was supported in part by grants from Ross

Laboratories, Johnson & Johnson, William R. Rorer, Inc., Sandoz Pharmaceuticals, Syntex Laboratories, Upjohn Company, CIBA Pharmaceutical Company, Merck Sharp & Dohme, Roche Laboratories, E.R. Squibb & Sons, Inc., Boehringer Ingelheim Ltd., and Geigy Pharmaceutical Company. However, this book does not necessarily reflect the opinion of the American Geriatrics Society, which was acting solely as a forum for the exchange of ideas, or of the supporting institutions.

This was also the first meeting of the Section of Teachers of Geriatric Medicine of the American Geriatrics Society. In addition to the major chapters in this book, there are a number of very short essays contributed, with one exception, by the audience of that meeting. They are included in the appendix. Just as not every major issue of geriatric medicine could be included, not every nuance of those chosen could be addressed. Nonetheless, I do want to take this opportunity to thank each participant in Chicago who spoke formally or informally, whether author or not, either behind or in front of the podium, for contributing to my understanding of geriatric medicine.

I would be remiss if I failed to thank a host of individuals who contributed substantially to this undertaking. William Reichel, M.D., deserves special commendation as he encouraged and nurtured the whole concept of a Section of Teachers of Geriatric Medicine. All other members of the Board of Directors of the American Geriatrics Society without a single exception, including those of the recent past, have invariably supported a variety of related educational developments as well as this particular book. Kathryn Henderson, Executive Director, and Marcia Roye, Associate Executive Director, have given me encouragement at every opportunity. This simple notation simply cannot convey the magnitude of my gratitude to them. With no sense that priority is dictated by order of appearance, Gretchen Batra, M.S., Charlotte Johnson, and Lisa Medoff, all of Boston University, deserve and have my most sincere appreciation for their organizational skills and extraordinary patience in the management of the Third Inter-University meeting and in compiling this book. Bernadine Richey of Collamore Press was invaluable as copy editor. Our thanks are found on every page. Finally, in order to be both timely and sound, the preparation of a book of this nature requires the skills and efforts of one very central figure. All of us were especially lucky that Mara Hardy assumed that role. Each of the authors owes her a debt of gratitude.

Knight Steel, M.D.

Note

1. This analogy was included in a paper delivered to the Committee on Geriatric Medicine, National Institute of Medicine, National Academy of Sciences, March, 1978.

Reference

1. Aging and Medical Education. Institute of Medicine. National Academy of Sciences, Washington, D.C.: September, 1978.

Contributing Authors

Ronald D. Bayne, M.D., F.R.C.P. (C), F.A.C.P.
Professor of Medicine, McMaster University, Hamilton, Ontario
Medical Services Consultant, St. Peter's Centre, Hamilton, Ontario

Owen W. Beard, M.D.
Professor of Medicine, University of Arkansas School of Medicine, Little Rock,
  Arkansas
Chief, Division of Geriatrics, Little Rock Veterans Administration Medical Center,
  Little Rock, Arkansas

David W. Bentley, M.D.
Associate Professor of Medicine, University of Rochester School of Medicine and
  Dentistry, Rochester, New York
Head, Infectious Diseases Unit, Monroe Community Hospital, Rochester, New
  York

Anna Bissonnette, R.N., M.S.
Assistant Professor of Community Medicine, Boston University School of Medi-
  cine, Boston, Massachusetts
Director of Patient Care, Home Medical Service, University Hospital, Boston,
  Massachusetts

Frank R. Brand, M.D.
Coordinator of Geriatrics, Clinical Campus/SUNY Upstate Medical Center at
  Binghamton, Binghamton, New York

Stanley J. Brody, J.D., M.S.W.
Professor of Physical Medicine and Rehabilitation in Psychiatry, University of
  Pennsylvania Medical Center, Philadelphia, Pennsylvania

Evan Calkins, M.D.
Professor of Medicine, State University of New York at Buffalo, Buffalo, New
  York
Head, Division of Geriatrics/Gerontology, Department of Medicine, Veterans
  Administration Medical Center, Buffalo, New York

Barbara Cahn, M.S.W.
Special Assistant to the Deputy Secretary
Department of Health and Mental Hygiene, State of Maryland

Jon C. Calvert, M.D., Ph.D.
Professor and Chairman, Department of Family Practice, Medical College of
 Georgia, Augusta, Georgia
Chief, Family Practice Department, Talmadge Memorial Hospital, Augusta,
 Georgia

Edward W. Campion, M.D.
Instructor in Medicine, Harvard Medical School, Boston, Massachusetts
Chief, Geriatrics Unit, Massachusetts General Hospital, Boston, Massachusetts

David K. Carboni, Ph.D.
Director, Center for the Study of Aging, College of Health Sciences, University
 of Bridgeport, Bridgeport, Connecticut

Rodney M. Coe, Ph.D.
Professor, Department of Community Medicine, St. Louis University School of
 Medicine, St. Louis, Missouri

James F. Conover
Member, Board of Directors, Union Hospital, Terre Haute, Indiana

Bess Dana, M.S.S.A.
Professor, Department of Community Medicine, Director, Education Unit,
 Mount Sinai School of Medicine of The City University of New York, New
 York, New York

Gerald R. Gehringer, M.D.
Professor and Head, Department of Family Medicine, Louisiana State University
 School of Medicine, New Orleans, Louisiana
Senior Visiting Physician, Charity Hospital New Orleans, New Orleans, Louisiana

Richard J. Ham, M.D.
Chief, Division of Geriatrics, Department of Family Practice, Southern Illinois
 University School of Medicine, Springfield, Illinois
Staff Physician, Department of Family Practice, St. John's Hospital, Springfield,
 Illinois

Antoinette M. Hays, R.N., M.S.
Assistant Professor of Nursing, Boston University School of Nursing, Boston,
 Massachusetts
Geriatric Nurse Practitioner, Geriatrics Section, University Hospital, Boston,
 Massachusetts

Sumner H. Hoffman, M.D., F.A.A.P., F.A.A.F.P.
Professor, Department of Community Medicine and Socio-Medical Sciences, Boston University School of Medicine, Boston, Massachusetts
Chief, Department of Community Medicine, Director, Home Medical Service, University Hospital, Boston, Massachusetts

Joseph H. Holtzman, Ph.D.
Director, Gerontology Center, Oklahoma University Health Sciences Center, College of Health, Oklahoma City, Oklahoma

Stanley R. Ingman, Ph.D.
Associate Professor of Family and Community Medicine, University of Missouri-Columbia School of Medicine, Columbia, Missouri
Director, Postdoctoral Program Mental Health and Aging, University of Missouri-Columbia, Columbia, Missouri

Jean E. Johnson, M.S.N., N.P.
Director, Adult and Geriatric Nurse Practitioner Program, George Washington University, Washington, D.C.

Robert L. Kane, M.D.
Professor of Medicine, UCLA School of Medicine, Los Angeles, California
Senior Researcher, Rand Corporation, Santa Monica, California

Lawrence J. Kerzner, M.D.
Assistant Professor of Medicine, Boston University School of Medicine, Boston, Massachusetts
Director, Geriatric Education Program, Jewish Memorial Hospital, Boston, Massachusetts

Hugo Koch, M.H.A.
Health Statistician, National Center for Health Statistics, Sterling, Virginia

Edward G. Lakatta, M.D.
Assistant Professor of Medicine, Johns Hopkins University Medical Institutions, Baltimore, Maryland
Chief, Cardiovascular Section, National Institute on Aging, National Institutes of Health, Baltimore, Maryland

Jonathan D. Lieff, M.D.
Assistant Clinical Professor of Psychiatry, Boston University Medical School
Director of Psychiatry and Geriatrics, Lemuel Shattuck Hospital, Boston, Massachusetts

Richard W. Lindsay, M.D.
Associate Professor of Internal Medicine and Family Practice, University of
Virginia School of Medicine, Charlottesville, Virginia
Head, Division of Geriatrics, Internal Medicine Department, University of
Virginia School of Medicine, Charlottesville, Virginia

Michelle L. Marcy, M.S.
Visiting Instructor, Department of Family Practice, Southern Illinois University
School of Medicine, Springfield, Illinois

John D. Murphy, R.N., M.S.
Geriatric Nurse Practitioner, University of Rochester School of Nursing, Ro-
chester, New York
Nurse Practitioner, Monroe Community Hospital, Rochester, New York

L. Gregory Pawlson, M.D., M.P.H.
Director, Center for Aging Studies and Services, George Washington University,
Washington, D.C.

Valery A. Portnoi, M.D.
Assistant Professor, Health Care Science Department, George Washington University, Washington, D.C.
Director, Geriatric Medicine Division, George Washington University, Washington, D.C.

Morton I. Rapoport, M.D.
Professor of Medicine and Senior Associate Dean, University of Maryland School
of Medicine, Baltimore, Maryland

Duncan Robertson, M.D., F.R.C.P. (C)
Associate Professor and Head, Department of Geriatric Medicine, University
Hospital, Saskatoon, Saskatchewan

John W. Rowe, M.D.
Associate Professor of Medicine, Harvard Medical School, Boston, Massachusetts
Director, Gerontology Division, Beth Israel Hospital, Boston, Massachusetts

Dennis J. Selkoe, M.D.
Assistant Professor of Neurology, Harvard Medical School, Boston, Massachusetts
Associate Neuropathologist, Mailman Research Center, McLean Hospital, Bel-
mont, Massachusetts

Ethel Shanas, Ph.D.
Professor of Sociology, University of Illinois at Chicago Circle, Chicago, Illinois

Richard P. Shannon, M.D.
House Officer, Department of Medicine, Harvard Medical School, Boston, Massachusetts
House Officer, Department of Medicine, Beth Israel Hospital, Boston, Massachusetts

Marcia R. Smith, Ph.D.
Visiting Instructor, Department of Family Practice, Southern Illinois University School of Medicine, Springfield, Illinois

Kenneth Solomon, M.D.
Assistant Professor of Psychiatry, University of Maryland School of Medicine, Baltimore, Maryland

Kevin R. Sorem, B.S., P.A.-C.
Geriatric Physicians Assistant, Division of Geratric Medicine, Department of Health Care Sciences, George Washington University School of Medicine and Health Sciences, Washington, D.C.

Knight Steel, M.D.
Associate Professor of Medicine, Boston University School of Medicine, Boston, Massachusetts
Chief, Geriatrics Section, Evans Memorial Department of Clinical Research and Department of Medicine, University Hospital, Boston University Medical Center, Boston, Massachusetts
Director, Gerontology Center, Boston University, Boston, Massachusetts
Chief, Section of Teachers of Geriatric Medicine, American Geriatrics Society

Franz U. Steinberg, M.D.
Professor of Clinical Medicine, Washington University School of Medicine, St. Louis, Missouri
Director, Department of Rehabilitation Medicine and Senior Attending Physician, Department of Medicine, The Jewish Hospital, St. Louis, Missouri

Lawrence T. Tremonti, M.D.
Associate Dean, Clinical Campus, SUNY Upstate Medical Center at Binghamton, Binghamton, New York

Robert E. Vestal, M.D.
Assistant Professor of Medicine, Divisions of Clinical Pharmacology, Gerontology and Geriatric Medicine, University of Washington School of Medicine, Seattle, Washington
Staff Physician and Coordinator for Research and Development, Veterans Administration Medical Center, Boise, Idaho

M. William Voss, M.D.
Assistant Professor, Department of Family Medicine, University of Maryland School of Medicine, Baltimore, Maryland
Director, Division of Geriatrics, Department of Family Medicine, University of Maryland Hospital and Harbor Health Care Center, Baltimore, Maryland

T. Franklin Williams, M.D.
Professor of Medicine, University of Rochester School of Medicine and Dentistry, Rochester, New York
Medical Director, Monroe Community Hospital, Rochester, New York

Carol Winograd, M.D.
Assistant Professor, University of California at San Francisco, San Francisco, California
Attending Physician and Chief, Geriatrics Program, Department of Medicine, San Francisco General Hospital, San Francisco, California

An Overview

1

Geriatrics for Educators and the Educated

Knight Steel, M.D.

In 1970 Freeman surveyed the catalogues of the 99 medical schools in the United States [1]. He determined that in less than half of them was there even a single citation about aging. Only 14 offered special courses in geriatrics or aging at a clinical level and most of these were offered by divisions of psychiatry, preventive medicine, or public health. An additional 10 medical schools included some geriatric training in general clinical courses, not one of which was offered by a department of medicine. Of the approximately 22,000 faculty at these 99 medical schools, only 15 were concerned specifically and primarily with aging, including those doing basic research. Notwithstanding the obvious difficulties encountered when drawing conclusions from a survey of catalogues, it does seem reasonable to maintain that little was happening in the field of geriatrics a decade ago.

Today, eleven years after the appearance of Freeman's article, geriatrics is a matter of considerable interest, and perhaps some measure of debate as well, at many schools of medicine. Unlike most medical school subjects, geriatrics can be viewed from a variety of quite-different vantage points by many medical specialties, including internal medicine, family practice, rehabilitation medicine, public health, and psychiatry. Furthermore, geriatric medicine is a matter of unique concern to many professions other than medicine, especially nursing, allied health, social work, and hospital administration, to many institutions, such as nursing homes, acute and chronic hospitals, and health maintenance organizations, and most especially to the government.

Within the more circumscribed medical community, however, certain events and dates of the 1970s stand out. A publication entitled "Recent Developments in Clinical and Research Geriatric Medicine: The NIA Role" [2] documents the very special place of this newest institute of the National Institutes of Health in the changes that have occurred during the last ten years. Drawing upon this publication and other resources, it is possible to note a few of the more important geriatric happenings of the 1970s.

In 1972, Libow established the first formal geriatric residency program in the United States at the Mt. Sinai City Hospital Center in New York [3]. The goals of his program were "to develop special clinical skills to deal with the

Dr. Steel receives support as a recipient of the Geriatric Medicine Academic Award (#1 K07 AG00060–01), National Institute on Aging, National Institutes of Health.

medical and psychosocial problems of the elderly and to achieve the ability to develop health care systems for the elderly." Individuals admitted to his program had two or three years of a standard internal medicine residency.

Four years later, in 1976, a conference focusing on geriatric medicine was convened in Washington, D.C. by the Institute of Medicine of the National Academy of Sciences in collaboration with the Royal Society of Medicine [4]. The program was notable for its highlighting of the geriatric program in the United Kingdom.

Interest in adapting the British experience to the American scene has been considerable. However, this may not prove to be easy or desirable. The National Health Service of the United Kingdom is a formal health-care system with both a large number of general practitioners and a very small number of geriatricians who act solely as consultants and care for a significant segment of the hospitalized and institutionalized aged. In striking contrast, the American health-care industry is notable for its lack of a system with doctors functioning independently in roles of their own choosing with respect to each other and to the patients they serve. There are no easy mechanisms to allow for the centralized planning of services to the elderly or for the allocation of resources.

Furthermore, there is considerable discussion in the British literature about the ability of geriatric medicine, as it is presently structured in the United Kingdom, to compete with other specialties in medicine for staff positions, money, and facilities [5,6,7,8]. Thus, although we should adopt the intent of our colleagues in the United Kingdom to improve the health care of the elderly specifically, we may find it impossible and indeed undesirable to copy the ways they have proposed to accomplish this end.

Exactly how geriatrics should be introduced into both academic medicine and the health-care system has been a matter of discussion for some time. In 1976 and 1977, the American Geriatrics Society, with support from the National Institute on Aging, invited a group of about thirty-five individuals, representing both professional societies and academic institutions, to two meetings to discuss the appropriate place of geriatrics in medical education [9]. A number of models for the teaching of geriatric medicine were presented. Most important, it was the consensus of the group that geriatrics should not be broken off as a discrete subspecialty but, instead, more effort should be directed toward infusing content about aging into both the medical school curriculum and the postgraduate years. For persons with a special interest in geriatrics, it was recommended that a residency or fellowship of one to two years might be developed as part of a traditional program in a recognized specialty, such as internal medicine, family practice, or psychiatry.

During the 1970s, the Veterans Administration established six, and more recently eight, Geriatric Research Education and Clinical Centers (GRECC) to promote geriatric research as well as service for its aging constituency [10]. In 1978, the Veterans Administration established a geriatric fellowship program at

12 of its hospitals. When fully operational, these programs will support 24 fellows at a first-year level and 24 additional persons in the second year.

A milestone occurred in 1977 with the establishment of the Irving Sherwood Wright Professorship in Geriatrics at the New York Hospital-Cornell Medical School. This was the first chair in geriatrics at an American medical school.

Also in that year, a committee of the Institute of Medicine, the National Academy of Sciences, was convened to collect information about the state of geriatric medicine and to suggest directions for its future [11,12]. They issued a report entitled *Aging and Medical Education,* in which they presented eight major recommendations:

1. Medical schools should include appropriate content on aging in basic and clinical-science courses. The establishment of a complementary required course that integrates knowledge about aging and the problems of the elderly is favored.
2. Preparation for the care of the aged should be included in clinical clerkships and in house-staff-training programs, as well as in examination for certification and licensure.
3. Nursing homes and other long-term-care facilities should be included in clinical rotations for medical students and house staff. Experience with home health programs and other alternatives to institutionalization is also desirable.
4. Teaching about aging should receive increased emphasis in continuing medical education (CME), and the Liaison Committee on Continuing Medical Education and its sponsoring organizations should support increased geriatric content in CME programs.
5. Medical schools should develop a cadre of faculty to teach gerontology and geriatrics to medical students and house staff. Postresidency training or fellowship programs should be developed in settings that have either the necessary leadership in geriatric medicine or have a potential for promptly developing it, and a limited number of career development awards in gerontology and geriatrics should be established.
6. The establishment of a formal practice specialty in geriatrics should not take place, but the recognition of gerontology and geriatrics as academic disciplines within the relevant medical specialties should be encouraged.
7. Efforts to meet the education needs of medical directors of skilled nursing facilities should be assumed jointly by medical schools and the nursing facilities.
8. Funding should be expanded in various aspects of aging research including the basic biological and behavioral sciences, clinical medicine, and health services research.

Reaction to these recommendations has been generally favorable. Some interested and informed persons contend that geriatrics must be recognized and accredited in a more formal manner. The arguments in favor of such a position include, on the one hand, the contention that there is today a body of specialized knowledge in the care of the elderly and, on the other, the belief that geriatrics cannot survive in academia without the political clout accorded it by board certification of one type or another. Most recently, the Association of Professors of Medicine issued a statement regarding geriatric medicine that is generally in agreement with the recommendations of the Institute of Medicine [13].

These, then, are the especially prominent occurrences of the 1970s that were instrumental in defining the state of geriatrics in the early 1980s. This listing of historical events does not recognize the great efforts of a number of individuals in the field who antedated these very-recent occurrences and who labored diligently, often in relative obscurity. Perhaps most notable in geriatric education was Frederick D. Zeman who offered a course in geriatrics in 1944 as part of a postgraduate teaching program at the College of Physicians and Surgeons, Columbia University, in New York [14]. His course consisted of sixteen lectures and emphasized

> a) the knowledge of the aging process and its effect on clinical manifestations; b) the physical and mental hygiene of old age and the prevention of disease; c) the importance of psychologic and psychiatric understanding; and d) the social and economic forces affecting the lives of the old.

The impact of these recent events and those that surely will take place within the near future has already, and will continue to have, a profound effect at three levels of medical education: the basic science years in medical school, the clinical years in medical school, and the postgraduate medical years. Let me discuss these in sequence.

Since the program for the first two years of medical school is usually rigidly controlled, and since even minor deviations from the proscribed format is a cause célèbre on curriculum committees, most geriatricians have targeted their efforts at revision of courses within the preclinical curriculum. It has been found to be easier to persuade the directors of each of the curricular units in the first two years, be it cell biology, physiology, pharmacology, or pathology, to include an appropriate amount of gerontologic material than it is to wedge a new course into an already overcrowded program.

If what is taught in these preclinical years is to be relevant to the medical student's upcoming experience, some basic knowledge should be proferred not only about the "ideal 70-kg man" but also about the "not unusual 80-year-old woman," who will, after all, more nearly typify the patient cared for in later years. Furthermore, such an approach can alter a faculty member's opinion about gerontology in a favorable way and may well facilitate the recruitment of new investigators into the field.

Sometime during these first two years, or occasionally at the very beginning of the third year of medical school, there is an essential yet long-neglected course concerned with history-taking and physical diagnosis. I would like to make a plea for the total rejuvenation of this course—perhaps by turning it over to the division of geriatrics in each medical school! To support this proposition, I would point out first that the patients in our teaching hospitals are aged. Last year at Boston University Medical Center, 45% of 200 consecutive admissions to two floors of a medical service were 65 years of age or over.[1] Thus, many of the patients in our university hospitals are being treated by house staff almost 50 years their junior. It is not surprising, therefore, that there are significant social and cultural differences between the caretakers and the persons being cared for.

Furthermore, it is widely recognized that the elderly individual frequently fails to present a "typical complaint"—"typical" as described in our textbooks of medicine. Additionally, the symptoms of many illnesses seen in the geriatric population are vague and nonspecific. Although the detailed information about each pathological entity should be imparted during the clinical clerkships, there must be an acceptance of more realistic norms for the process of history-taking by both faculty and students. Some might argue that it is for reasons of good pedagogy that classical examples of classical diseases are preferentially displayed in history-taking courses; however, the nature of what is classical is questionable as vague symptoms and difficult-to-tease-out complaints become increasingly commonplace.

The case for management of history-taking courses by the division of geriatrics is supported by a review of texts of general physical diagnosis [15]. A survey of eleven such books, including those suggested for most medical students in the United States, revealed not one reference to geriatric care. It was rare that even a single sentence commented on how to take a history from someone hard of hearing. Detailed examples of histories were presented by the authors but on only one occasion was the patient portrayed as being over 65 years of age.

Elderly individuals often have multiple complaints. In order to adequately evaluate such cases, sufficient time must be allocated to the task of history-taking and considerable skill must be employed in separating one complaint from another. Regrettably, only a single text acknowledged the concept of multiple chief complaints.

Furthermore, each book surveyed assumed that a hospital or, less frequently, a clinic was the setting for the interview. Not a single one offered the possibility that the setting would be a nursing home or chronic-disease hospital. Yet, there are now about 1.2 million long-term-care beds in the United States, a number larger than the number of acute-care hospital beds. About one in five of all Americans of all ages will pass through such institutions at one time before death [16]. Surely many physicians must take histories in these surroundings. Also, it is not unusual for the student to be advised to describe a typical day in the life of the patient at the end of the written history. Never have I seen described in an acute hospital chart a typical day in a nursing home!

Most medical schools retain the third-year clerkship in medicine, surgery, pediatrics, psychiatry, and perhaps, obstetrics and family practice. In the rotation on the medical service, a student is expected to gain further skills in history-taking and physical diagnosis together with the fundamentals of medical management. Traditionally, this component of the third-year curriculum has been considered central to the education of all medical students, regardless of what branch of medicine each selects to enter at the end of the fourth year.

Although the acquisition of clinical knowledge and skills and the adoption of a humane attitude are each essential to the final product of our educational system, it is the latter area of concern that merits special attention. Although a humane attitude most surely has been in the process of development since childhood, it is not unreasonable to believe that such attitudes are shaped to a significant degree during the third-year clerkships by exposure to role models and through direct experience. It is, therefore, a matter for concern that Spence et al. reported more negative attitudes toward the elderly among senior students than among freshmen [17]. In this regard, Gale and Levesley quote a British medical student as saying "We come to clinical medicine with humanity and after three years they have educated it out of us" [18].

Faculty must concern themselves with why older patients especially are labeled with derogatory names, even if by exhausted house officers. Regrettably, this may occur with the tacit complicity of faculty who may feel inadequate to manage persons who have multiple interlocking illnesses within the purvue of half a dozen subspecialties.

Only slightly less pernicious is the habit of describing patients as "interesting," for that implies that some, usually the aged, are not interesting. Thus, rounds with the professor take place more often in a conference room than at the bedside and concern themselves with an especially "interesting" patient, which is usually translated to mean a person afflicted with only one disease and that the one the professor is expert on. The principles of management taught often imply a thorough, if poorly thought out, diagnostic workup and an attempt to control the disease in an acute hospital setting.

As noted, an older patient often reflects a complex of diseases and multiple social problems, which collectively prevent the individual from being fully functional. Besides exceptional skill in history-taking and physical diagnosis, the management of such persons requires an understanding that most of their diseases are chronic conditions and, more importantly, that they must be cared for over time. This requires a rather extensive understanding of the multiple pathological conditions, a knowledge of what is normal for older persons, the nature of any expected interactions among the multiple conditions and among their therapies, and some appreciation of what sociocultural circumstances contributed to the present decompensated state and how they may be addressed, either at home or at some lower level of care. These "uninteresting," usually geriatric, patients on our medical service offer an exceptional opportunity for stimulating discussion.

Therapeutic interventions in the elderly individual also promise many chances for clinical satisfaction. A patient with multiple medical and social difficulties can be returned to a markedly improved state of functioning not only by one but by any number of and many types of intervention. Third-year medical students must be taught that medicine cures little except acute infectious illnesses. Thus, the older patient often represents a great opportunity to practice clever and sophisticated management of both disease and social ills. The establishment of the "Most Uninteresting Patient Rounds" or, more formally, "Geriatric Rounds," on every medical service might allow for the appropriate discussion of such truly fascinating patients.

Concern with education for clinical care in no way detracts from the need for geriatrics to be viewed by third-year medical students as a partner in clinical investigation with the subspecialties of internal medicine as well as neurology, psychiatry, rehabilitation medicine, and health-care research. The special knowledge and unique skills of these other specialties will be essential to assure clinical advances in geriatrics.

The fourth year of medical education has become a collection of electives. Departments of medicine traditionally offer two kinds of rotations. The first is an acting internship, often demanding in time and energy but considered to be of experiental value for the rising house officer; the second is a subspecialty consulting rotation, often less demanding in time and energy and considered exciting because it is tutorial in character. Programs in geriatrics have begun to offer both the classic types of electives and others as well.

A few academic institutions have designated a small number of beds in the acute hospital as a geriatrics unit where elderly persons are evaluated. In the United Kingdom, this practice of establishing a discrete geriatric ward is not unusual. Perhaps more likely to become a permanent part of our health-care system in America is the development of geriatric units at chronic-disease hospitals or high-level skilled nursing homes.

The inclusion of long-term-care facilities in teaching programs makes it possible for students and faculty to work with both highly skilled and relatively unskilled health-care professionals and to recognize the importance of the latter, often poorly educated and poorly motivated, to the well-being of the patients. Students and faculty will come to understand which medical situations can be managed effectively in such facilities and which cannot. The success of these educational ventures depends on attracting students and that depends on making the quality of care at these long-term-care institutions first rate and the quality of the faculty the same [19].

It remains an embarrassment to the profession of medicine that it is still possible, and indeed likely, for a physician to become a board-certified internist after a minimum of eight years of professional training without ever once having seen a long-term-care patient. Generals are said to complain that battles are always fought at the edge of their maps. So faculty trained in acute-care hospitals will have to see to the edge of their experience and beyond if they are to perform their duties as teachers of what is important for the care of all patients.

A consultative service in geriatrics will compete for students with other traditionally popular consultative services. This part of the geriatrics program might also be operated in conjunction with general medicine. The consultative service established within the Department of Medicine at Boston University Medical Center is unique, to my knowledge, in that a geriatric nurse practitioner is the initial professional to respond to the request for consultation. Following her extended visit with the patient, during which she takes a history and performs a physical examination, a detailed evaluation is made by the doctor. A consultation form is completed by both nurse and doctor making use of other health professionals, especially social workers and physical therapists, where needed, and suggestions are made about medical and nursing care, rehabilitation efforts, and placement, as required.

Few programs that include an experience in the delivery of home care to the elderly have been established by departments of medicine, although collaborative efforts with other academic divisions, especially family practice, are being considered. Those programs that do exist offer students, and even house officers, a better understanding of how many of our patients live as well as the profound effect cultural and socioeconomic factors have on their state of well-being.

As clinical geriatric units become operational, offering one type of experience in the tertiary care-setting, another in a long-term-care institution, and perhaps a third in home care, it will become more commonplace to have house staff spend a portion of time on a geriatric rotation. At least one month (3% of the three postgraduate years now required for internal medicine) should be allocated to a mix of experience in chronic hospitals, nursing homes, and home-care settings. Initially, such rotations may not be popular with house staff, but much of the negative feeling could be overcome, in my opinion, by more appropriate faculty attitudes and a serious commitment to the ideals of geriatric medicine on the part of the departments of medicine [20,21,22].

In keeping with the recommendations of the National Institute of Medicine, a number of fellowships in geriatric medicine have been established. Each tends to draw on whatever strengths were in existence prior to its beginning. Thus, there are geriatric fellowships that emphasize metabolic or neurologic research and there are those that might more appropriately be viewed as postdoctoral programs in biochemistry. The danger of many of these fellowship programs is the tendency to pattern the fellowship so closely on the program already in existence that nothing new is produced other than one additional fellow in a recognized subspecialty. Furthermore, the striking variability is likely to create some difficulty for the house officer who is applying for the post and who might not recognize that each geriatric fellowship program is quite so individualistic. However, this variation does allow for exceptional opportunities for training in the research skills of an array of specialties.

If all of the educational efforts in geriatrics in the medical school and during the postgraduate years succeed, what will academic medicine have accomplished? Unquestionably, today's programs will produce investigators of all types. Some will be neurogeriatricians, others will be cardiogeriatricians. It is to be hoped that students will enter the field of long-term-care for purposes of both service and research, but all physicians will understand more clearly the phenomenon of aging and what that process means to our physiologic reserves and our adaptive responses to injury and infection. Every physician will gain more insight into a patient's diseases, needs, and functional state because every physician will have better skills for physical assessment, know more pathophysiology, and be more compassionate through a better understanding of aged persons. Every physician will know more about clinical pharmacology and other therapeutic modalities and how to utilize those resources available for coping rather than curing and for caring over time. Such physicians will then be elegant physicians.

Note

1. Data compiled as part of a study, Hospital Occurring Iatrogenic Illnesses, carried out by K. Steel, P. Gertman, C. Crescenzi, and J. Anderson (NIH grant No. 5 R21 AG01178-01).

References

1. Freeman, J.T. A survey of geriatric education: Catalogues of United States medical schools. *J. Am. Geriatrics Soc.* 19:746, 1971.

2. *Recent Developments in Clinical and Research Geriatric Medicine: The NIA Role.* NIH Publication No. 79-1990. August 1979.

3. Libow, L.S. A geriatric medical residency program, a four-year experience. *Ann. Intern. Med.* 89:641, 1976.

4. Exton-Smith, A.N., Evans, J.G. (Eds.). *Care of the Elderly: Meeting the Challenge of Dependency.* New York: Gruen & Stratton and London: Academic Press, 1977.

5. Leonard, J.C. Can geriatrics survive? *Brit. Med. J.* 1:1335-1336, 1976.

6. Cross, V.H. Geriatric medicine—death and rebirth. *Brit. Med. J.* 2:816, 1977.

7. Medical Care of the Elderly. Reprint of the Working Party of the Royal College of Physicians of London. *Lancet* 1:1092, 1977.

8. Harrison, J.F. Geriatrics and medicine: Both sides of the fence. *Lancet* 1:866, 1978.

9. Reichel, W. (Ed.). Proceedings of the American Geriatrics Society, Conferences on Geriatric Education. *J. Am. Geriatrics Soc.* 24:481, 1977.

10. U.S. Government. *Report on the Aging Veteran.* 95th Congress, 2nd Session, Senate Committee, Print No. 12. Washington, D.C.: Government Printing Office, January 5, 1978.

11. Institute of Medicine. *Aging and Medical Education.* National Academy of Sciences, Washington, D.C.: 1978.

12. Dan, P.E. and Kerr, J.R. Gerontology and geriatrics in medical education. *N. Engl. J. Med.* 300:228, 1979.

13. Statement of Professors of Medicine, 1979.

14. Zeman, F.D. Teaching geriatrics: Basic principles and syllabus of course now in fifth year. *J. Ger.* 4:48, 1949.

15. Steel, R.K. A clinical approach to communication with the elderly patient. In L. Obler and M. Albert (Eds.), *Language and Communication in the Elderly: Clinical, Therapeutic, and Experimental Issues.* Lexington, Mass.: Lexington Books, D.C. Heath and Company, 1980.

16. Harris, C.S. (Project Director). *Fact Book on Aging: A Profile of America's Older Population.* Washington, D.C.: National Council on the Aging, Inc., 1978.

17. Spence, D.L., Feigenbaum, E.M., Fitzgerald, F., and Roth, J. Medical students' attitudes toward the geriatric patient. *J. Am. Geriatrics Soc.* 16:976, 1968.

18. Gale, J. and Livesley, B. Attitudes toward geriatrics: A reprint of the King's survey. *Age and Aging* 3:49, 1974.

19. Clark, D.W. and Williams, T.F. (Eds.). *Teaching of Chronic Illness and Aging.* Bethesda, Maryland: National Institutes of Health, 1973.

20. Leaf, A. Medicine and the aged. *N. Engl. J. Med.* 297:887, 1977.

21. Beeson, P.G. Training doctors to care for old people. *Ann. Intern. Med.* 90:262, 1979.

22. Butler, R.N. Geriatrics and internal medicine. *Ann. Intern. Med.* 91:903, 1979.

Clinical Resources
and Facilities

2 Introduction

T. Franklin Williams, M.D.

The aim of this section is to discuss the wide range of settings in which the clinical aspects of geriatrics take place. We should keep in mind that clinical geriatric teaching, to be fully adequate, must include experience in every type of environment in which older persons are likely to need care. The requirements of geriatric patients are varied: some need ambulatory preventive and maintenance care, some need the social and health supportive services of home-care systems and institutions of varying types, and some need hospital care. In turn, the characteristics of these environmental settings influence the way in which care is given.

The chapters that follow illustrate the wide variety of settings in which the teaching of geriatrics takes place for medical students, house staff, nurses, nurse practitioners, and others. A number of conclusions emerge:

1. Successful teaching can go on wherever there is a good teacher; conversely, no matter how appropriate the setting, without a good teacher it will not be effective.

2. Most of the developments to date in the use of various settings and facilities for geriatric teaching have been opportunistic and spotty. That is, a medical school may have developed good teaching in a long-term-care setting because of interests and ready availability but may not have developed any home-care teaching. Another medical school may have done the reverse; while still another may have concentrated on ambulatory geriatric teaching. It is doubtful that a comprehensive teaching program that incorporates all of the settings in which elderly are cared for exists in any of our medical schools at present. Thus, efforts by medical schools to become more comprehensive are important. At the same time, however, it makes sense for a medical school to give special attention to its strongest possibilities.

3. There is the need to distinguish between the teaching of medical students and the teaching of house staff. In some settings, geriatric programs have approached these two groups as an undifferentiated entity even though their levels of development and career commitment are different.

4. There is an intense need for new knowledge in geriatrics, as a basis for ongoing substantive and exciting learning. This applies to knowledge that needs to be derived from basic research, clinical research, epidemiological research, and the evaluative research of new health-care programs for the elderly. The view has been expressed that most of us who are now teaching geriatrics, who our-

selves are relatively new to the field, have in the past few years "caught up" on the knowledge available and now find only limited amounts of substantial new knowledge being added. This is typical of any new field of learning but highlights the importance of vigorous research and scholarship.

5. As we approach a design for geriatric teaching, we should start with the geriatric patient wherever he or she may first be seen, determine that patient's needs, find the necessary services, and care for the patient in the variety of settings that may be called for over time. This includes looking for new alternatives for care that may not initially exist in a given community. This approach should apply both to our care of elderly patients and our approach to teaching geriatrics.

6. We should make a specific effort to include other health professionals by adopting a systematic approach for choosing and involving other health professionals, not simply by leaving it to chance.

3 Geriatric Teaching in the Clinic

Richard W. Lindsay, M.D.

Health care for the elderly must be personal and highly individualized. This is extremely difficult to achieve in many of our traditional teaching clinics. Dr. Francis Weld Peabody pointed out some of the problems related to training and teaching in these settings when he said, "the primary difficulty is that instruction has to be carried out largely on the wards and dispensaries of hospitals, rather than in the patient's home or physician's office" [1]. We are all aware of the need for more "well" geriatric or noninstitutional experiences for our residents, as well as the need for stronger training in the care of the institutionalized elderly population. Yet, for the most part, we persist in utilizing the institutional setting as the sole training site for our residents.

Part of the problem is due to the fact that residents have only one option— to institutionalize their patients. There is no funding for home care and we have not developed appropriate alternatives. We urgently need more day-care facilities, after-care programs, home-care programs, and other noninstitutional settings to allow for the appropriate interdigitation of care perhaps centered on some occasions in our teaching clinics.

There exist tremendous opportunities for geriatric teaching in a clinic setting under the auspices of the University Primary Care Internal Medicine Residency Program. For example, residents usually have little experience in rehabilitation, the assessment of activities of daily living, geriatric prescribing, the socioeconomic problems of geriatric patients, geriatric dental care, podiatry, and the workings of the community health-care system. I have found the residents not only responsive but extremely interested in all these areas.

Mention of the community health-care system also serves to point up a major problem that exists in geriatric teaching in most university hospital primary-care practices. That problem is the lack of any strong link between the community, with its home-care system, and the teaching practice. Dr. W.F. Anderson said, "services for the elderly must be community-based since most older people wish to remain in their own home for as long as possible" [2]. Therefore, resident physicians receiving geriatric training must know how to utilize these community-service networks and any home resources that are available.

Another problem related to community health care is the lack of faculty who are comfortable in the home or community setting. As departments of community medicine have declined or actually disappeared, family practice programs have often been asked to assume the role of the community-training programs, even though they also have faculty problems. Hopefully, our renewed interest in the elderly and the increase in the number of geriatric fellowship programs will produce teachers who can and will function as role models in clinic, community, and home settings.

I have made another observation about teaching in the university primary-care setting. That is, that professionals from other disciplines so necessary for optimal geriatric patient care, are seldom found within the confines of the teaching clinic. Therefore, it is extremely difficult to exchange information about patients, or to inform the resident in some detail, about the talents and capabilities of the other professionals.

Before leaving the clinic setting, I want to say a few words about the "team" in geriatric health care. Unfortunately, like geriatric faculty, there are very few examples of functioning interdisciplinary geriatric health-care teams in our medical training sites. I tend to agree with those who feel that the concept of a health team is a figure of speech. I feel strongly that if the next generation of physicians is to play an effective role in geriatric health care, then the scope of their experiences and training in the interdisciplinary group setting must be expanded, as well as their knowledge about nonmedical and psychosocial areas.

It is apparent that family practice has led the way at many universities towards more comprehensive health services for the elderly. They have also been the pioneers in the training of young physicians in the psychosocial and socioeconomic areas of medical care. At the University of Virginia School of Medicine there is now much greater emphasis on the teaching of psychosocial material in the primary care internal medicine program. I think this is a direct result of the influence of the university's family residency program. Family practice training programs also are involving residents in home health care through home visits. Model units are excellent places for geriatric teaching; however, I think that we will need the output of all training programs that are oriented toward primary care, such as internal medicine, psychiatry, and family practice, if we are to answer the needs of the geriatric patient as well as the overall needs of the country.

One should also consider the private practitioner's office as a setting for geriatric teaching. In my experience, this is a most appropriate arena for the delivery of optimal service to the elderly patient. The doctor-patient relationship in this setting is unimpeded by long delays and other problems inherent to university clinics. Many private physicians have mastered the team-care approach. They have learned which individuals in the community can be used as resources in the management of their elderly patients at home. They understand the use of the third-party financing system to optimize patient-care resources. More important, they have learned the value of home nursing and the family as resources in geriatric health care. They also have included the wishes of the patient and the patient's family in the care prescription. These latter three points must become major goals for our residency training in geriatrics.

My experience has been that the practicing physician's office, when used as a preceptorship setting, can be an extremely effective site for the training of residents. I feel we should utilize it whenever possible, and we are currently doing this in a rural setting for our primary care/internal medicine residents and family practice residents at the University of Virginia. One rural practice has an associated nursing home that further assists us in our geriatric training program.

In designing this unit, it is anticipated that the program for an ambulatory geriatric facility at the University of Virginia will become the focus for all geriatric services in this area. We plan to utilize a multidisciplinary medical staff with appropriate representation from the specialties of dermatology, urology, orthopedics, psychiatry, neurology, internal medicine, rehabilitation, dentistry, and podiatry. At the same time, we plan to integrate portions of all agencies responsible for the delivery of services to the elderly in the Charlottesville area and place them in the same facility with this interdisciplinary medical team. These services include the area agency on aging, the senior centers, the Meals on Wheels program, the local bar association, home nursing, the local transportation network, and the local government. We will also draw upon other major university resources, such as the Schools of Business and Architecture, for additional talents that can be made available to our senior citizens.

We hope that by centralizing all these individuals and services in the same location, we can immediately facilitate service to our elderly citizens, but more important in the long run, we will be able to enhance the transfer of information between the various members and residents and students in training. A major effort of this group will be the education of families and other individuals responsible for the care of the elderly patient. We will also have a geriatric inpatient facility located at the same site. We have been helped in our program design by the location of the Departments of Psychiatry and Neurology at this physical site. A major rehabilitation effort is also being located here with a plan to include day care, after care, and hospice care. This site will then become the major laboratory for the training of medical students, residents in the primary-care disciplines, nursing students, and other health professionals.

References

1. Peabody, E.W. Care of the patient. *JAMA* 88:877, 1927.
2. Anderson, W.F. Geriatric medicine—The challenge of the 1970's. *S. Afr. Med. J.* 50:1218, 1976.

Home Care as a Site for Geriatric Teaching—The Experience at Boston University

Sumner H. Hoffman, M.D.

Home care for the elderly is being recommended as a comprehensive solution to the increasing institutionalization of the geriatric population of this country [1]. While we are not prepared at this time to promote home care as a universally comprehensive and cost-effective alternative to long-term institutional care, we believe that for a majority of patients, especially those who have not reached the "greatly impaired" level, it is a cost-conscious and cost-effective system of health care that certainly improves the quality of life of the partially impaired, housebound geriatric patient. For these and other reasons, home care should be a site for geriatric education.

The University Hospital Home Medical Service has a long-time teaching commitment to the students at Boston University School of Medicine. It was in 1875 that the physicians of the Free Clinic associated with the Massachusetts Homeopathic Hospital began this home-care program. As the need for service increased, additional personnel were added and historical figures indicate that up to 7,000 house calls were made in a single year. After Boston University School of Medicine affiliated with that hospital, medical students were allowed to participate in the program. Massachusetts Homeopathic Hospital became Massachusetts Memorial Hospital and then University Hospital, which in turn joined with the Boston University Schools of Medicine and Graduate Dentistry in the establishment of the Boston University Medical Center. The affiliated Schools of Nursing, Social Work, Allied Health Sciences, and Law and Management made available a spectrum of capabilities for the comprehensive teaching of the problems of delivery of health care in the patients' homes.

Although the program has always been family oriented, originally concerned especially with pediatric and obstetrical care, it now emphasizes geriatric medicine. Furthermore, the overwhelming use of lying-in facilities for obstetric care eliminated the need for home deliveries and the advent of the neighborhood health centers in the early 1970s, with pleasant, readily available care for children, left the service with a predominantly homebound elderly population. The Home Medical Service reassessed its role at this time and became the principal purveyor of geriatric home care in the core city area of Boston.

The present day catchment area includes the most striken areas of Boston as well as the affluent areas of Beacon Hill and encompasses a population of about 170,000 people. Using the population demographic data collected by the

Health Systems Agency and the Area Agency on Aging, 13% of this population are 65 years of age or older, giving a potential target population of about 23,000.

Currently the Home Medical Service has an enrolled patient load of over 700 individuals who require comprehensive care. Several hundred additional patients who are "actively inactive" are seen only on the basis of need and in an episodic fashion. According to a report to Congress [1] by the Comptroller General of the United States, published in January, 1978, about 17% of those 65 or over fall into the greatly or extremely impaired category and about 33% of those in this category are in institutions. Applying these bench marks to our projected elderly population of 25,000, some 4,200 are extremely impaired and 1,400 of these should be expected to be in nursing homes or other long-term-care institutions. We have not broken down our served population by degrees of infirmity but an educated guess would place 30% to 40% in the greatly impaired category.

In order to encourage continued mobility, the Home Medical Service maintains and operates nine mini-health centers in elderly housing units in various parts of the city. The Boston Housing Authority and Section VIII housing developers, such as State Street Development Corporation of Boston, have assisted our efforts by making apartments available for our clinic activities. We have provided the necessary medical equipment and personnel and, in some cases, even the furniture.

Patients using walkers, crutches, wheelchairs, and canes are encouraged to obtain their maintenance care at these clinics and are seen in their homes when their infirmities periodically preclude clinic visits. A further extension of our care includes a three-morning-a-week clinic at University Hospital for patients who attain a greater degree of mobility. This clinic allows patients to be brought in by van or ambulance for tests or examinations that are difficult or impossible to perform in the home, for example, pelvic examinations, radiologic and ultra-sound studies. The physicians of the Home Medical Service have admitting privileges at University Hospital and thus provide continuity of care to their patients when hospitalization is needed.

Offices of the Home Medical Service are maintained at Boston University Medical Center in the Doctors' Office Building where one division of the Boston Visiting Nurse Association, composed of eighteen staff nurses, share office space and conference rooms. Our staff consists of three full-time physicians, three part-time physicians who provide a half-time equivalent, four nurses, one of whom is a registered nurse practitioner, four social workers and three secretaries.

The multidisciplinary approach to health care which characterizes our service will be discussed in another chapter; however, I will describe the medical student involvement on the Home Medical Service.

This rotation is a one-month requirement for all fourth-year students at Boston University School of Medicine with the only alternative option being a family practice preceptorship, to which approximately 33% of the class is assigned. Each month, six to eight students are divided into three teams, each with a physician preceptor, nurse, and social worker. Commencing July, 1980, residents from the Department of Medicine at University Hospital began rotating through the Home Medical Service as part of a larger obligatory geriatric medicine rotation, bringing a new dimension of geriatric education to the hospital house staff. Home visit or mini-clinic assignments are made, and the teams are deployed each afternoon to their designated areas. An average of 450 patient visits are made monthly. Supervision of the students' work is the responsibility of the team physician, who discusses the various facets of patient care on site with the students or at case conference the following day. At morning conference, the full staff meets with the students of the various teams to hear presentations on the new patients who were seen the previous day, a brief summary of revisits to patients made without the benefit of preceptor supervision, and problem cases or cases of special interest to the entire group. Patients seen with the preceptors are not reviewed. Care plans are evolved, social service needs are discussed, and therapeutic regimens are established.

Following case conference, a geriatric lecture series has been established with a one-hour daily presentation by Boston University staff members from various disciplines and specialties. Included in this series are such subjects as financing of health care for the elderly, sexuality, law and medicine, and patient's rights, as well as more traditional yet pertinent medical material as afforded by the various subspecialties. Once a month, in collaboration with the Geriatric Section of the Department of Medicine, geriatric grand rounds are held.

Problem-oriented records are maintained, and students are expected to participate in the hospital care of patients they have admitted to the University Hospital under the care of preceptors. An innovative concept of record keeping, advocated by Dr. Theodore Reiff of North Dakota, which he calls the life medical history [2], is being considered as the most valid way to accumulate chronological data without losing resolved problems, which can have implications for health care years later.

The goals of this program are to:

1. Introduce the students to the principles of geriatric medicine.
2. Demonstrate the various methods of establishing support services to maintain the elderly in their home environment by utilizing community agencies.
3. Identify the strengths of family and other caretakers as an alternative to institutionalization of the severely disabled elders. (An excellent paper on this subject was published by Callahan, Diamond, Giele, and Morris [3].)
4. Develop an awareness of home, environmental, and social factors as determinants of the wellness of the elderly population.
5. Allow the student to gain an understanding of the problems of dementia, depression, and mental health in the population, an ability to recognize the

relationship between them, and an appreciation of the use of remotivational programs to improve or delay the tendency to withdraw or disengage from society.

6. Demonstrate the use of the multidisciplinary health-team approach to the care of older people.
7. Permit the student the opportunity to become aware of the increasing problems inherent in long-term-care institutions by visiting them.
8. Instruct the student in the problems of degenerative diseases, multiple diagnoses, and atypical reactions of the elderly to acute illnesses and therapeutic agents.

While these goals are designed for the University Hospital Home Medical Service, they are universal in concept and can be applied to any teaching program that has a medical school affiliation.

An important consideration for all geriatric programs is the means of funding them. The Home Medical Service was supported in the past by grants from various private foundations (Commonwealth Fund, Clark Foundation) and federal agencies. Currently, however, the program receives funding for educational activities from the medical school with the rest of its support for direct patient care coming from University Hospital. Since we are part of the ambulatory services of the Department of Medicine, billing for physician visits to the homes and clinics and for the daily care of patients in the hospital is accomplished by the business office of the hospital at rates established by the Massachusetts rate-setting commission.

Almost all of our patients are insured through the Title XVIII Medicare program with a large majority also eligible for Medicaid Title XIX benefits. Indeed, our social workers often are called on to implement applications for Medicaid benefits for patients who were unaware of their eligibility. A small number of patients are privately insured, and a still smaller number have no insurance. In the latter case, the hospital has reduced charges, or, in isolated cases, waived the charges incurred by their care. Only those visits made by a staff physician-preceptor are billed to the third parties; there are no charges made for student visits. Between 20 and 30 of our patients are hospitalized at all times. With this source of income to the hospital, plus the collected fees, our service is economically sound.

While this program is geared to a core city urban model, it would be possible to extend it to a more affluent population if waivers could be obtained to increase the Medicare home visit reimbursement formula. Certainly it is cheaper to pay for home visits by a physician than for daily acute hospital care.

Although we believe the Boston University School of Medicine/University Hospital Home Medical Service is the oldest continuous home-care program in this country, I would like to call attention to the fact that other excellent home-care programs exist that can be used for teaching purposes. Special attention should be directed to the Montefiore Hospital Program as well as other alternative programs, including geriatric day-care centers, geriatric specialized housing, and nursing programs established as hospital-based, coordinated, home-care agencies. Dr. Rossman has enumerated and described these in detail in his chapter in *Clinical Aspects of Aging,* edited by Reichel [4].

References

1. Home Health—The Need for a National Policy to Better Provide for the Elderly. *Report to the Congress* by the Comptroller General of the United States. December 30, 1977. Published January 1978.

2. The Life Medical History Evaluation and Care of the Geriatric Patient. Dr. Theodore Reiff, Professor of Medicine, Director, Institute of Gerontology and Geriatrics Medicine University of North Dakota, Personal Communication 1979.

3. Callahan, J., Jr., Diamond, L., Giele, J., and Morris, R. Responsibility of families for their severely disabled elders. *University Health Policy Consortium* (Boston University, Brandeis, MIT), July, 1979.

4. Rossman, Isadore. Newer options for the elderly patients other than institutionalization. In W. Reichel (Ed.), *Clinical Aspects of Aging.* Baltimore, Md.: Williams and Wilkins, 1978.

Health Maintenance: An Awareness of the Importance of the Home, and the Health-Care Team —Three Principles Addressed in a Home-Care Setting

Anna Bissonnette, R.N., M.S.

This chapter deals with only three of the eight objectives identified by Sumner Hoffman, M.D. in chapter four. These objectives are the ones that, in my view, form the foundation for all the others. They are:

1. Introduce the students to the principles of geriatric medicine.
2. Develop an awareness of home, environment, and social factors as determinants of the wellness of the elderly population.
3. Demonstrate the use of a multidisciplinary health team approach to the care of older people.

Principles of Geriatric Medicine

This objective receives the lion's share of time and energy in the program. Efforts are directed to as many facets of geriatric care and as many aspects of gerontology as time will allow. One aspect of geriatric medicine is the need to understand the difference between *health maintenance* and *crisis intervention* and the importance of the former in the care of the elderly. Hickey, in his monograph, *Health and Aging,* comments that ". . . regardless of the setting or care option selected, there are two generic forms of health care that must be considered when planning for the elderly. They are *intervention* and *prevention*" [1]. Intervention is direct care in response to an actual problem. In this country's medical-care system, which is a "sick-care" system, intervention predominates.

Prevention, on the other hand, occurs without the belief or knowledge that something is wrong. The first goal of prevention is the avoidance of onset of disease. In a population that is beset with many chronic conditions and a diminishing physiological reserve, prevention is harder to accomplish than treatment and rehabilitation. What is called secondary prevention is concerned with "slowing down" the disease process once it has begun, thus preventing the occurrence of complications and a future deterioration of function.

Over the years the Boston University Home Medical Service staff has developed a model for service that has attempted to address this principle of prevention, both primary and secondary, and health maintenance. Therefore, once a patient has been accepted for service and given as full an assessment as possible, a schedule for regular monitoring is established. Students contact the patient and alert the individual to the need for a check-up, although the point is made that in home care, as always, the patient has the right to accept or reject the services.

The Home Environment and its Impact on the Wellness of the Elderly Population

We are seeing a significant redefinition of what "home" means to an older person. When this service considers "home," it realizes that "regardless of how humble a dwelling may be, the integrity and privacy of this sanctuary for each patient must be defended and supported so long as it is rational." It further dictates that an individual has the right to the dignity of dying quietly at home, protected from the hospital scene and all that that represents.

The Health-Care Team

The use of a health-care team is, in my opinion, an approach by which health-care professionals put aside traditional expectations of medical care hierarchy, each professional thereby having equal say in patient care decision making. Philip Brickner, in his book, *Home Health Care for the Aged*, describes the milieu for successful team functioning as an egalitarian one [2]. Not any one problem, be it medical, social, nursing, or other, can, strictly on the basis of professional category, be of a higher order than the others and thus automatically reflect one professional's decision-making prerogative. This is in contrast to the traditional pattern where medical problems tend to be the most important and, therefore, physicians are expected to be chief decision makers.

Margolis, in an article discussing changing disease patterns, states: "The basic characteristics of an American health care system are not conducive to an approach which envisages geriatric care at a comprehensive primary care level, within a system of health care, combining medical and social activities in a team led by a competent physician. Since such an approach seems to be a most appropriate one, an attitude on the part of the medical profession which concentrates on the medical aspects only and neglects the entire complex of problems, substantial and organizational, associated with geriatric care, may lack utility" [3].

An attempt to implement an effective team approach is embodied within the activities of the Home Medical Service's approach to primary health care of the elderly. Teams are composed of a physician, nurse, social worker, several medical students, a physician's assistant student, a pharmacy student, and a nurse practitioner student. As noted by Hoffman, teams meet formally each day at a case conference, during which detailed presentations are made for team consultation, and a care plan is drawn up. Once the care plan has been agreed on, the delineation of tasks for its implementation takes place and the more informal network of communication and follow-up is set into motion. It is through this process of communication and coordination that the complex problems of our clients are attacked, and the special skills of our staff are utilized. Students of all types are directly involved in this process so that each will understand better what the other health-care providers on the team have to offer the patient, the family, and the community at large.

References

1. Margolis, E. Changing disease patterns, changing values: Problems of geriatric care in the U.S.A.–an outsiders view. *Medical Care 17*:1119, 1979.

2. Brickner, P.W. *Home Health Care for the Aged: How to Help Older People Stay in Their Own Homes and out of Institutions.* New York: Appleton-Century-Crofts, 1978.

3. Hickey, T. *Health and Aging.* Monterey, California: Brooks Coles Publishing Company, 1980.

The Use of a Geriatric Evaluation and Placement Service as a Resource for Teaching

Ronald D. Bayne, M.D.

No component of health care is more influenced by cultural and political standards and expectations than a system that aims to assess holistic needs and to identify and coordinate services for long-term care. Therefore, in discussing evaluation and placement as a teaching resource, one should show not only the basic principles of assessment of the patient's needs, but also some basic approaches to finding and using resources. Teaching at the undergraduate, postgraduate, and, to some extent, practicing professional levels must be theoretical and practical. Education without training in the "real world" is relatively useless. Teaching should occur where the problems are normally found, and the learners should be involved in problem solving. This is important because health-care-delivery practitioners are involved in highly individualistic situations, which can be very different from the controlled setting of university teaching centers.

The objective of an evaluation and placement service is to help individuals, who have a range of health problems and disabilities, gain access to the health-care resources appropriate to their needs. To do this it is necessary to identify their needs and remaining abilities as well as their expectations and wishes, to identify the resources that can be used to meet these requirements, and to facilitate admission when necessary. A placement service can also monitor the actual use of resources, guide health professionals in using and developing resources, and identify deficiencies in resources for the use of health planners.

Opinions vary as to how evaluation and placement services should be organized. Some geriatricians believe that virtually every elderly person with long-term-care needs should be assessed by a specially trained team. Some believe that a health screening clinic is necessary to find elderly persons with needs not yet identified. Some placement services identify resources needed but have no authority to gain admission; others have exclusive authority over access and can assure the individual of admission to a facility deemed appropriate by that placement service.

The Assessment and Placement Service (APS), established in 1971 in the Hamilton Wentworth Health District by the District Health Council [1], is pragmatic and continually evolving. It serves a population of approximately 500,000, of whom approximately 40,000 are aged 65 or more. There is a rich array of health services ranging from four teaching hospitals, ambulatory clinics, a mental hospital, several chronic hospital core facilities and a variety of long-term personal-care facilities to a home-care program with short-term and long-term options. Costs of care for all of these resources are covered in whole or in part by the Health Insurance Program. Other resources, such as lodging and boarding homes, senior centers, senior citizen housing and family social services, are also available.

The patient's needs are assessed by the patient's personal physician, along with a nurse and social worker if in a hospital or a community nurse if at home. The information is recorded in two parts on a standard form. A nurse counselor in the APS office scans this information, identifies the type of care and service required, and recommends one or several placements to the physician and patient or family. The use of the service is voluntary, but it would appear that over 80% of patients in institutions are placed through this service. There are about 2,000 referrals annually. Time lapse from referral to placement varies greatly depending on urgency and availability; there is a caseload of over 700 persons. Because of the complexity of each case and the large case load, the basic information is held in a computer data bank for review and updating.

The APS form is repeatedly modified in the light of use and criticism by its users. It is standard in that one form is used for all referrals to APS, but it has not been tested for inter-rater reliability. The form provides basic data, but more detailed information can be added as required. In addition to asking for information about the applicant, the form asks what placement the physician, nurse, and social worker desires, although the final recommendation is based on the type and degree of incapacity shown. Follow-up after placement has demonstrated that the information is accurate in most cases, and the placement is reported as satisfactory for over 90% of those persons investigated.

The educational role of the APS has been extensive. Initially, it was necessary to convince physicians and other professionals that more detailed assessment was needed and that placement location mattered! It was necessary to show the various resource facilities that the information provided by the APS was accurate enough for them to use with confidence. It was necessary to show the public that such a system had advantages over a system where influence and political pressure were keys to access. Let me say that in the cultural and political reality in which we work, we do not claim to have achieved complete success; however, we have the opportunity of being heard by the practicing professionals who are asking for help.

The system has enabled health professionals to provide reliable information, although they still appear not to understand what services various facilities can and cannot provide. They seem to perceive all chronically disabled persons as one indistinguishable group. To overcome this, we are developing a system of categories, each of which identifies a different program of treatment or care. A category contains a group who share certain characteristics that distinguish them from all others. The characteristics chosen are those that describe needs and relate to specific services or programs of care. Obviously, chronically ill and disabled elderly persons have complex needs and can belong to several categories. However, such categories make the purpose of placement clear, and the type of care that will be needed more readily discernable. Being asked to identify a category for patient care helps health professionals to understand more clearly how the care needs of each patient relate to an appropriate facility.

The APS system, indeed any evaluation and placement system that is concerned with all types of patients and all types of resources, provides the tools and methods for improving and monitoring placement and long-term care. It is a valuable resource for teaching how to ask the significant questions in assessment, how to communicate with other professionals who will provide ongoing care, and what kinds of constraints and concerns nonteaching institutions frequently manifest.

The Teaching of Geriatrics in an Acute Hospital Setting

Knight Steel, M.D.
Antoinette Hays, R.N., M.S.

When the teaching of geriatric medicine is discussed, considerable emphasis is usually placed on the use of long-term-care facilities in training programs, the need for the multidisciplinary approach, and the necessity of including both healthy elderly persons and home-bound patients in the experience of medical students [1]. All of these points are important, and each reflects an aspect of geriatric medicine that is essential to the development of a comprehensive program of education. However, the vast majority of training time for both medical students and housestaff is spent on the wards of acute-care hospitals and this is unlikely to change in the near future. If geriatrics is to compete effectively with other clinical specialties, it must develop a component of service in the acute-care setting. In order to accomplish this, a division of geriatrics could develop a discrete geriatric unit and/or a consultative service. Let us consider these two options, beginning first with a discussion of a geriatric ward.

An inpatient geriatric ward might resemble one of the following three types of units presently in existence. First, there is the unit designed to provide a special service, which is multifactorial in character. This variety is typified by the coronary-care unit and the intensive-care unit with the relatively unique access to monitoring equipment and the well-trained nursing staff. A geriatric unit based on this model would provide overall service not readily available elsewhere in the hospital. It is difficult, however, to determine what unique factor or group of services would warrant the establishment of such a unit, at least as a part of a medical service. Furthermore, it must be remembered that between a third and a half of all patients on the Medical Service of our tertiary care hospitals are 65 years of age or over. Assuming that the unit was not so large as to comprise almost half of all the medical beds, we must consider which of the medical patients would be on a geriatric unit, managed by acute hospital standards and reimbursed at hospital rates. That is, which among our elderly patients would require the unique services of a geriatric unit and, perhaps more importantly, which should be excluded from such a unit.

The most obvious benefit of a discrete unit, especially of this type, is that it could be staffed and administered in such a way as to respond to the special

Dr. Steel receives support as a recipient of the Geriatric Medicine Academic Award (#1 K07 AG00060), National Institute on Aging, National Institutes of Health.

needs of the elderly in the same way, for example, that oncology units respond to the special needs of the cancer patient. However, if we are to learn from the experience of departments of geriatrics in the United Kingdom, such units all too often become the place for patients who are simply difficult to discharge [2,3]. This can be true under a system where inpatient and outpatient services are coordinated and function under the control of a single individual. The American health-care system under present circumstances operates in striking contrast to such an organized system of care. Furthermore, the English experience has pointed up the difficulty in staffing and in maintaining the moral of the staff on geriatric wards.

A second kind of inpatient facility that can be considered as a prototype for a geriatric ward is typified by the endoscopy unit. Usually the *raison d'etre* of such units is a special procedure or a very specialized need. Patients may not even be officially transferred to such units, remaining there for only a part of a day, or they may be admitted directly from home for a short stay, ranging from a few hours to a few days. Some hospitals have holding areas attached to emergency rooms where patients are admitted who require a procedure not able to be carried out in a clinic setting. It seems difficult to adapt this type of a unit for geriatric use as geriatrics has no monopoly on a type of tube or catheter. Also, when it is anticipated that an elderly person will be admitted to a hospital for only a brief stay, the kinds of services likely to be required are quite different from those most persons would envision on a geriatric unit. As a rule, persons admitted for a mix of medical and social reasons (a common occurrence in geriatric medicine) are rarely discharged home or to a lower level of care after only a few days in the hospital. On the other hand, it is possible that a respite-care unit could be modeled to some extent on a short-stay ward. Third-party payment mechanisms need to be established before respite care can be implemented to any significant degree in the United States.

A third type of inpatient unit on which a geriatric unit might be modeled is the research unit where service is not the prime consideration. It certainly would be possible to establish a geriatric research unit or geriatric metabolic ward. If, however, the patient had an illness requiring the kind of monitoring demanded by most clinical research protocols, it seems both costly and unwise to pursue a separate clinical research unit for the elderly. Furthermore, a unit designed to study the many chronic problems associated with old age is justifiable but not at acute hospital reimbursement rates. Such a geriatric research unit could be established at a chronic hospital as long as invasive or potentially harmful procedures were restricted to those for which adequate care was available should a problem arise.

Perhaps the most compelling argument in support of a discrete geriatric unit is that it allows for a significant measure of power for geriatrics within the academic structure. Some might argue *sotto voce* that this is so critical a consideration for geriatrics that, notwithstanding contradictory arguments of merit, geriatrics should pursue its own group of beds for teaching and service. Perhaps the recent history of the struggles of departments of family practice supports this contention. In balance, however, the establishment of such walled-off units can harm the development of geriatrics in the future for they run the risk of falling victim to many of the problems experienced by our colleagues in the United Kingdom. In addition, discrete units segregate the elderly from the mainstream of medicine whereas the geriatric patient population has almost become the mainstream itself.

Although the concept of separate and distinct geriatric wards may be difficult to support, the principles of geriatric care exemplified by such units should prevail in the care of all elderly patients on the medical service and indeed on other services as well. The implementation of these most worthy objectives might better be accomplished in an acute-care hospital by means of a geriatric consultative service.

Patterned to some degree after the consultative service operated by the subspecialties of internal medicine, such a geriatric consultative service could respond to requests to see patients throughout the hospital. The single major drawback for a consultative service as a teaching tool is that it might not be asked to consult—no small consideration! Before returning to this critical issue, I will assume for the moment that this would not be the case and will comment on the advantages of a viable consultative service.

First, this type of program would allow the division of geriatrics to influence care throughout the hospital. Since the geriatric staff will be quite limited in size and stamina for the foreseeable future, a consultative program will maximize the exposure of both medical personnel and nursing staff to the teachings of the geriatric program. In addition, one or more senior medical students, house officers, or fellows could have a rotation on the geriatric consultative service just as they presently do on the cardiology or hematology consultative services.

Second, such a service would permit professionals from the subspecialties of internal medicine, together with those from neurology, psychiatry, rehabilitation medicine, nursing, social work, and the allied health professionals, to collaborate in the care of a single elderly person. Rather than having a series of unconnected consultations added to the chart, this one service would attempt to manage all needs of the patient, especially, but not limited to, those persons admitted to the surgical subspecialties. Where necessary, the geriatric service would consult with other specialties whose advice in turn would influence the management of the patient being seen by geriatrics. This seems to be an exceptionally fruitful way to learn how to deliver care.

Third, as has been suggested by Leaf [4], our medical services need a role model in geriatric medicine. What better way to provide it!

The prime disadvantage of a consultative service, as has been noted, is that geriatric medicine might not be asked to see enough patients to warrant its use for teaching purposes. Although this is undoubtedly possible, requests for consultation will be received if the service provided is found to be helpful by others.

Since a nurse would be a part of the consulting team, the geriatric consultative service would work closely with the nurses on the floors. Since the nursing service plays an increasing role in the day-to-day management of many elderly persons in acute hospitals, it is not unreasonable to expect that house officers will be encouraged by the nursing staff to request help from geriatrics where appropriate.

This brings us to two further issues about a proposed consultative service. First, what type of patient is an appropriate one for geriatrics to see? It might be expected that geriatrics will be requested to visit persons who cannot be placed. This is both true and not unreasonable, for a geriatrician could point out, for example, that a nursing home would be much more willing to accept the patient if something could be done about the patient's incontinence. Other patients for whom a consultation might be sought are those suffering a change in mental state, especially if it occurs in the hospital setting, or those who are simply "failing" with multiple problems. Also, consultations might be sought for older persons undergoing surgery. The geriatrician could clear the patient for the operation and suggest ways to limit the duration of confusion that might be anticipated to follow surgery. Geriatricians might see elderly patients who are both psychiatrically disturbed and physically ill, help manage them in the hospital, and plan for their care following discharge. Knowledge about and access to beds at one or more lower levels of care might be helpful in the management of some of these patients and might be a special contribution by a geriatric team with liaison to other health-care facilities and social agencies in the community.

The method of payment is another issue to be raised about a geriatric consultative service. Whether sufficient numbers of consultation requests will result in an adequate reimbursement for time expended by the team is unclear. We would point out, however, that this problem is not unique to geriatric medicine but is shared by many consultative services, such as those offered by infectious disease or endocrinology units. Furthermore, innovative ways to support this service, which might be quite effective at limiting health-care costs, might be arranged.

In November 1979, a consultative service was introduced at University Hospital, Boston University Medical Center, by the Geriatric Section of the Department of Medicine. The objectives of this service are:

1. to respond to the specific request of the referring physician,
2. to address the total health care needs of the patient while in the hospital, and
3. to consider what options are available for after-hospital care and facilitate the transfer of the patient out of the hospital to an appropriate level of care, be it home, nursing home, or a chronic hospital.

At the present, this geriatric service receives about three consultation requests per week, which (as a point of comparison) places it approximately between the Nephrology Unit and the Arthritis Unit in activity. No formal notification of the program was made initially except that the service was announced to nursing supervisors at the hospital at the time of its inception. The initial response to a request for consultation is made by a geriatric nurse practitioner, then the patient is seen by an internist with a special interest in the elderly, and a three-page consultation form is completed and signed by both individuals. When necessary, collaborative action occurs with other medical specialties or, more frequently, other types of health-care professionals. Follow-up visits by physician or nurse are made when indicated.

The reasons given for requesting a consultation were varied but it is our impression that many consultations were ordered by the physician because the Geriatric Service offered suggestions about total care. This was true for consultations not only from the Surgical Services but from the Medical Service as well. Involvement with the Nursing Service on the floors has been extensive. Indeed, on a number of occasions nursing staff have been responsible for the request being made by the house officer.

Furthermore, many of the reasons, explicit or implicit, for consultations seemed to be matters within the expertise of the service requesting help. Thus, Medicine sought advice about generally failing patients, Psychiatry asked us to see patients admitted for suicide gestures, and Orthopedics requested advice as to how to manage a patient after an orthopedic procedure.

Senior medical residents (PGY-3) and geriatric fellows have begun obligatory rotations in the Geriatric Service. Medical and nurse practitioner students have also had experience on the consultative service. Although it is too early to judge this consultative program either as a service or as an educational tool, the following general comments might be made.

First, in spite of the limitations imposed by a very small staff, geriatrics has had a wide exposure at University Hospital. Second, the Geriatric Service has had an impact on patient care. This can be demonstrated at many points along the clinical continuum. Thus, new and important diagnoses have been made, therapy has been instituted or changed because of recommendations about drugs and rehabilitative services, and many patients' post-hospital options have been widened because of the dissemination of information about other institutions and services and the movement of patients to our long-term-care beds and to home with support. It is hoped that such a dramatic impact on such a wide variety of patients cannot help but be noted and appreciated by students at all levels.

References

1. Clark, D.W. and Williams, T.F. (Eds.). *Teaching of Chronic Illness and Aging* Bethesda, Maryland: National Institutes of Health, 1973.

2. Leonard, J.C. Can geriatrics survive? *Brit. Med. J.* 1:1335, 1976.

3. Medical care of the elderly. Reprint of the working party of the royal college of physicians of London. *Lancet,* 1:1092, 1977.

4. Leaf, A. Medicine and the aged. *N. Engl. J. Med.* 297:887, 1977.

Medical Education Opportunities Offered by Long-Term-Care Institutions

Lawrence J. Kerzner, M.D.

Offering a well-supervised experience in the delivery of health care in a long-term-care institution can provide great benefits to the training programs of medical students, house officers and fellows. Recommendations have been made that long-term-care institutions be included in clinical rotations for medical students and house staff [1]. Long-term-care institutions currently provide health care to more than 1.2 million people in the United States [2]. While only 5% of the elderly population live in such facilities at any one time, some 20% can expect to spend some time there. For most physicians in training, the long-term-care setting, and the strategies used in caring for those patients are completely unfamiliar [3]. Even though there are more long-term-care beds than acute hospital beds, house officers have little experience in developing the appropriate attitudes, skills, and knowledge necessary to manage the complex intertwining of problems of the people who reside in chronic-care facilities. That continuing medical care can be delivered on an inpatient basis as well as in the clinic, that it must be accomplished in the framework of a health care team, that all persons, especially those in long-term-care institutions, may have limited goals and constricted life styles which may be well accepted by these individuals, that there are specific skills needed to relate to the chronically ill elderly, and that high quality health care can be delivered outside of an acute tertiary care hospital—all of these concepts can be introduced.

Pointing out the numerical pressures and projected statistics about people residing in long-term-care facilities is frequently not sufficient to convince those involved in medical education about the importance of continuity of medical care in an inpatient setting. Physicians in training are aware of the benefits of continuity of care through their experiences in hospital outpatient departments. There they are eager to participate in providing medical care over time and enjoy assuming primary responsibility, under appropriate faculty supervision, for the regular care of their patients. Medical care given in long-term-care institutions is simply another one of many ways in which ongoing care can be provided, especially for those whose physical, social, or psychological needs are not met in noninstitutional settings [4]. A resident's preexisting values are broadened by combining an experience in long-term institutional care and possibly home care with their standard inpatient and outpatient experiences [5]. This also introduces the house officer to the idea that the responsibility of being an advocate for each individual patient extends over a long period of time. This may encourage positive attitudes towards managing multiple health problems of chronically ill patients and elderly patients in general.

There is no ideal situation where patient problems can be rectified and a state of wellness established, especially in elderly patients who may be compromised by a decline in organ function and a limitation of their functional reserves. Institutional living arrangements may be necessary when a multiplicity of problems are present that require the skills of multiple health-care team workers. The ability to function as a member of the coordinated health-care team is integral to effective functioning by the physician in almost any patient-care setting. While the physician should be the team leader under most circumstances, such an individual frequently is not the most important member of the group as that role may be assumed by nurse, therapist, or social worker. As compared to acute-care hospitals, attention in chronic settings can be directed to ongoing problems, since the press of continually arriving, acutely ill patients is not an ever-present feature, and the constant push towards short hospitalization is less pronounced.

Because limited goals are acceptable and appropriate to patients whose life styles are constricted by chronic illness, slow improvement, stabilization, or even slowing the progression of a disease are likely to be viewed as a therapeutic success. Learning what goals are realistically acceptable and leading the team towards them is an important skill that can be learned and then applied in other patient-care settings. Because caring for the chronically ill requires the physician to be concerned not only with disease but also with the patient's relationship to the disability, the members of the patient's family, and the community, the physician in training is made aware of the importance of the social and psychological factors involved in patient illness [6]. Acquisition of knowledge of specialized communication techniques, especially necessary with elderly patients, is fostered.

Ongoing assessment of patients' medical problems and functional limitations provides the physician in training with an opportunity to evaluate the appropriateness of patient placement and determine when different supporting services are necessary and where and when to institutionalize patients who can no longer be cared for at home. Effective use of the multiple levels of the institutional settings available for patient care can thus be taught. This may be helpful in reversing the trend that has allowed the hospital to become the center of health care for the elderly [7], even though older persons may not tolerate acute hospitalization well. The artificial distinctions among levels of care that long-term-care institutions are forced to adhere to by third-party paying agencies will be seen as bearing little relationship to the real needs of people.

The unfolding of pathophysiological events over time can be closely scrutinized in long-term-care settings, since the slower pace allows time for more careful attention to detailed management of problems with less than major physiological import. Of course acute and significant changes must be identified and dealt with rapidly and effectively [8].

An especially important feature that long-term-care facilities offer for medical education is that students do not have to compete with hordes of faculty, residents, interns, and other students usually present at classical teaching centers for a place at the bedside [9]. Students are real contributors to patient care in such facilities, and this may tend to foster even greater interest and concern. Charismatic and committed teachers are needed to effectively compete for students with the more "high powered" specialties at acute hospitals. In addition, house officers respond to a physician's duty as teacher by demonstrating clinical skills [10] and infusing new thoughts about patient management, which will improve the quality of care delivered by other professionals and paraprofessionals.

Currently, there are no provisions in third-party payment schedules to defray the costs of operating high-quality teaching programs at long-term-care facilities. This is a major impediment to the establishment of teaching programs at chronic-care institutions. Money invested to this end would be well spent as the final product would be practicing physicians who can make effective use of various sites and resources for delivering medical care. This is a major area for third-party payers to invest in for future efficiency [1].

Important new dimensions can be added to house officer training programs by involving students in the care of persons in long-term-care institutions. As Romano states, "the continued responsibility of the care of a chronically ill person adds immeasureably to the education of a physician and provides indispensible preparation for the work he is to do" [11].

References

1. *Aging and Medical Education.* Washington, D.C.: National Academy of Sciences, September 1978.

2. Somers, A.R. The nations health issues for the future. *Ann. Am. Acad. Polit. Soc. Sci.* 399:160, 1972.

3. Steel, K. *The Development of Geriatrics in a Department of Medicine.* Paper presented to the National Institute of Medicine, National Academy of Sciences, March 1978.

4. Williams, T.F. Staffing problems in long-term care. *Medical Care Supplement* 14:85, May 1976.

5. Leaf, A. Medicine and the aged. *N. Engl. J. Med.* 297:887, 1977.

6. Rodstein, M. (Chairman, Committee on Undergraduate and Continuing Medical Education of the Clinical Medicine Section of the Gerontology Society). A model curriculum for an elective course in geriatrics. *The Gerontologist* 13:231, 1973.

7. Portnoi,V.A. Health care system for the elderly. *N. Engl. J. Med.* 300:1387, 1979.

8. Williams, T.F., Izzo, A., and Steel, R.K. Innovations in teaching about chronic illness and aging in a chronic disease hospital. In D.W. Clark and T.F. Williams (Eds.) *Teaching of Chronic Illness and Aging,* DHEW Pub. #(NIH) 75–876. Bethesda, Md.: Government Printing Office, 1973.

9. Welter, D.J. Georgia plan for medical education in long-term care. *South Med. J.* 68:1353, 1975.

10. Lawson, I. The nursing home medical director—A new breed of mentor. *Geriatrics,* 31:91, 1976.

11. Romano, J. On those who care for the sick. *J. Chronic Disease* 1:695, 1955.

Medical Education at the Monroe Community Hospital: A Long-Term-Care Setting—One Student's Experience

Richard P. Shannon, M.D.

The embryonic state of curriculum development in this evolving field and the inherent complexities of education outside of the university hospital system in no way minimizes the need for training in chronic disease and disability in the long-term-care institutions, which have remained outside the mainstream of the medical care system for so long. The fundamental question remains whether the long-term-care setting is appropriate for the purposes of clinical education, and if so, what the fundamental components of this educational experience might be.

As a fourth-year medical student, I recently had the opportunity to participate in an elective in geriatric medicine at the Monroe Community Hospital (MCH), a chronic disease hospital and major teaching affiliate of the University of Rochester School of Medicine and Dentistry [1]. The following are observations on the viability and effectiveness of the training from the perspective of a "senior consumer" of medical education. The MCH is a 634-bed chronic disease hospital, which provides the complete range of long-term nursing needs (skilled, intermediate, and residential) as well as the rehabilitation and short-term acute needs of residents. The medical staff includes full-time faculty of 13 in medicine, 2 in neurology, and 3 in rehabilitation medicine, as well as 50 part-time faculty members from psychiatry and surgical subspecialties.

The bulk of the advanced medical clerkship in chronic illness and aging is concerned with a 35-bed acute medical unit. The unit is organized to provide care to residents and patients from other areas of the hospital and other chronic disease institutions who develop new acute illnesses or suffer exacerbations of long-standing diseases. It is staffed by two teams consisting of a first- and second-year resident and a senior medical student on an elective basis. Supervision and consultation is provided on a monthly rotation by a full-time faculty member. The medical team is called by the nursing or medical staff to evaluate problems that arise throughout the institution. The team then decides whether transfer to the medical unit is necessary for further diagnosis or therapeutic intervention. If it is decided that appropriate intervention can be implemented without transfer, the team makes recommendations and provides follow-up in a consultative capacity. Transfer is arranged if the condition warrants further investigation, and the patient comes under the care of the medical team to which he is admitted. The medical unit then is the focus for medical, neurological, and rehabilitative evaluation and provides, as appropriate, the interface between medical, social services, and other professional assessment.

The elective experience for medical students revolves around the theme of patient care. It emphasizes the need for unbiased observation and patience in history-taking when difficulties are encountered because of a patient's significant sensory impairments. The elderly patient is generally a wealth of physical findings, which allows one to sharpen the skills of physical diagnosis. In addition, appreciation of the elderly patient's milieu underscores the importance of not only physical but functional assessment, both as an indicator of disability as well as a parameter by which to assess therapeutic efficacy.

Consistently, the information generated by such a thorough examination was overwhelming and confusing and not readily applicable to a reductionist concept. New signs and symptoms could refer to several organs, and the classic presentations of textbook medicine were often altered or blunted by the superimposed aging process. The challenge of unraveling the atypical manifestations of illness occurred during teaching rounds, which were held three times a week. For the students, teaching and management rounds were supplemented by a series of didactic sessions in which germane topics were presented. This process made me more comfortable in dealing with confused patients and wiser in the use of potentially harmful procedures, such as the insertion of Foley catheters. From the initial evaluation, the goals of diagnosis and therapy were mitigated by concern for the patient's quality of life and were formulated accordingly. This required an understanding of this quality as it existed within the institution. The experience did much to allay my fear of institutions, previously perceived as prisons without any possibility of a fulfilling life. I observed many residents functioning well within the limits of their disability and at levels that were unattainable outside such a supportive environment.

There are certain unique features in the organization of this particular educational experience that deserve some comment. In my opinion, these characteristics of the program at the MCH illustrate the distinction between care in the acute hospital setting and a unique system of care that is more nearly typical of geriatric medicine.

First, the patient load assigned to the medical team is significantly less than that on a general medical floor in an acute-care hospital. As such, the pace is conducive to a thorough investigation of complex multiple pathologies. Time is available for spending one hour on an initial evaluation, as well as for making careful daily follow-up observations. Time is allocated for critical reading and discussion of areas of interest as well as problems. Also, the time necessary to make appropriate functional and quality-of-life assessments is not compromised by the traditional hectic pace of acute hospitals.

Second, the presence of full-time faculty members with an interest in aging and clinical geriatrics establishes a tone that lends credibility and professional acceptance to such a system of care.

Finally, the modalities of treatment in long-standing irreversible disease are seen to be less dependent on the hardware of medical technology than they are on interaction with the disciplines of rehabilitation medicine, psychiatry, and social service.

No doubt, each medical school is geographically located in reasonable proximity to a long-term-care institution, at which an educational program can be implemented. Such a program requires several ingredients to insure a high-quality educational experience in geriatric medicine. They may be divided into four groups.

Fundamentals of the Program

1. Facilities must be available to develop the skills of observation and integration of knowledge in the context of patient management.
2. Faculty with an interest in aging processes must be present to direct and teach certain topics in which competency will be required.
3. Curriculum development must include time for didactic sessions to insure that fundamental issues are covered.
4. Clinicians should be available to ensure that issues of quality of life guide all diagnostic and therapeutic endeavors.

Practical Considerations

1. Sufficient time must be available to balance patient care with instruction.
2. Support services in both medical and other health professions must be available to provide comprehensive care.

Scholarly Activities

As dictated by faculty interests, ongoing clinical studies (as was true at MCH) will add a scholarly element to the discussion of issues in aging.

Institutional Commitments

It is essential that the program have the genuine support (resources and personnel) of administration and academic departments, particularly medicine, psychiatry, and physical medicine and rehabilitation.

No doubt, such programs do not develop *de novo* and will require appropriate planning, collaboration, and imagination. With these principles in mind, these experiences will be well received by students, who will sense the commitment and understand its importance.

Reference

1. Williams, T.F., Izzo, A., and Steel, R.K. Innovations in teaching about chronic illness and aging in a chronic disease hospital. In D.W. Clark and T.F. Williams (Eds.) *Teaching about Chronic Illness and Aging.* DHEW Publ. # (NIH) 75-876. Bethesda, Md.: Government Printing Office, 1973.

10 The Veterans Administration Hospitals as Resources for Geriatric Education—The Experience at the University of Arkansas

Owen W. Beard, M.D.

The Veterans Omnibus Health Care Act, which became law on October 21, 1976, directed the Veterans Administration to:

1. Emphasize treatment programs particularly suited to meeting the health-care needs of an aging population.
2. Emphasize the education and training of health-care personnel specializing in the treatment of elderly persons and diseases and infirmities characteristic of an aging population.
3. Emphasize biomedical and health-service research designed to ameliorate geriatric-care problems.
4. Develop specific plans for meeting the special architectural, transportation, and environmental needs of an aging population.

Thus, the Congress of the United States has mandated the Veterans Administration to be prepared to deliver excellent medical care to our aged veterans.

Regardless of what age one uses to define geriatrics, Veterans Administration Hospitals have a significant number of eligible veterans over the age of 65 years: 2.97 million in 1980 and this number will increase to 8.05 million by 1995. Over 50% of all U.S. males over the age of 65 will be veterans by 1986 and by about 1990 this percentage will increase to 60%. Furthermore, the fact that there are well over 100 Dean's Committee hospitals testifies to the already significant involvement of Veterans Hospitals in medical student and postgraduate medical education and in biomedical research.

There is a second consideration that emphasizes the importance of Veterans Hospitals as a resource for geriatric education. Geriatrics in this country is awaiting a definition. Without getting into the argument of what ages and what level of care falls within the field of geriatrics, there is no single health-care system in this country that can match that of the Veterans Administration for its many levels of health care. With the exception of domiciliary care, almost all levels of care can be given by or through each Veterans Administration Hospital. Ambulatory care via outpatient clinics, hospital-based home-care programs, and nursing-

49

home care through the Contract Nursing Home program are available to almost all VA Medical Centers. Many have VA nursing homes and/or intermediate-care beds associated with the more traditional hospital wards and intensive care units. Thus, the system has the patients and all levels of health care for its geriatric patients. The only problem is deciding which part of this should be used as resources in geriatric education.

There is still another consideration that emphasizes the importance of Veterans Hospitals as resources for geriatric education. Almost all agree that delivery of optimum health care to geriatric patients requires a team effort. The smallest team might include a physician, nurse, and social worker, but a really effective health-care-delivery team requires many more members. Here again, the resources of a Veterans Medical Center can enrich geriatric care and geriatric education since the following health-care disciplines are represented in most VA Hospitals: medicine, nursing, social work, physical therapy, occupational therapy, speech pathology, dietetics, clinical pharmacology, dentistry, theology, geropsychiatry, public health nursing, and podiatry. Indeed, individuals representing all of these disciplines are members of our own geriatric team. Add nursing students, medical students, interns, residents in medicine, geriatric fellows, dietetic interns, communication pathology students, social work interns, rehabilitation medicine students, and others, and you have an active geriatric education program.

Let me describe how we have pulled all the above resources together into a functioning educational unit where geriatrics is organized as a division of the Department of Internal Medicine of the University of Arkansas School of Medicine and the Medicine Department of the Little Rock VA Medical Center. We have a 10-bed Geriatric Evaluation Unit as a part of the Medicine Service in an acute general medical and surgical hospital. Geriatric patients are admitted to this unit either directly or as transfers from the acute bed services for complete evaluation in order to identify all of their treatable problems. Every patient is evaluated by physicians, a geropsychiatrist, nurse, social worker, and dentist. Other team members participate in the evaluation process as indicated. Junior medical students, two interns, one medical resident, and one geriatric fellow are usually assigned to the unit. Attending rounds are made three times per week. All team members meet one morning per week in a teaching discharge-planning conference at which time each member presents the results of his evaluation and the team sets further disposition and treatment goals.

Patients who need longer rehabilitation or convalescent care are transferred to our 28-bed Geriatric Rehabilitation Unit. Approximately 66% of the patients in this unit are discharged to home care after an average stay of nine to ten weeks. This unit is used at present for the training of geriatric fellows, nursing students, communication pathology students, social work interns, and dietetic interns. A teaching discharge-planning conference is held at this unit also one morning per week, at which time rehabilitation and disposition goals are evaluated and set.

We assume responsibility for furnishing primary health care to all patients accepted into the division. Thus, we have a geriatric ambulatory clinic which meets two days per week. Our goal is to bring together all available family and community resources needed in the care of each elderly patient and, hopefully, to stabilize the patient in a home environment. Clinic patients are followed at intervals appropriate to each patient's needs. The social workers, nurse practitioners, and physicians who see patients in the ambulatory clinic are the same familiar faces who met the hospitalized patient.

An important part of our activity is our telephone reassurance program. The patient and their families are encouraged to call a specific phone number and talk to the nurse practitioner who has seen them both in the hospital and in the clinic, and ask about anything which is of concern. This program has resulted in fewer missed clinic appointments and a decrease in the number of unscheduled or emergency admissions to the hospital. We have approval for a Geriatric Day Care Hospital, but this has not as yet been funded. The Geriatric Division does not administer but does utilize the facilities of the Hospital Based Home Care Program and the Veterans Administration Nursing Home.

In summary, Veterans Administration hospitals represent a superb resource for geriatric education. They should be increasingly incorporated into the new and expanding programs at American medical schools.

Role of Veterans Administration Hospitals as Bases for Academic Units in Geriatric Medicine —A Historical Perspective

Evan Calkins, M.D.

In the previous chapter, Dr. Beard summarized several characteristics of the Veterans Administration system that can be used in the development of academic programs in geriatric medicine. Dr. Beard also illustrated how these assets can be utilized in the development of a teaching program by describing the experience at the Little Rock Hospital. My perspective is that of a newcomer to the system. Although I have served as a consultant to the Veterans Administration for the past nineteen years, it has only been during the last two years that my office and the largest segment of my program have been located within this system. I would like to share with you what I have learned about the history of the development of the Veterans Administration's interest in and commitment to long-term care, and then to add a few comments. I gratefully acknowledge my indebtedness to the staff of the VA office of long-term care for contributing to my knowledge, on this topic, but stress the fact that the perspective I present is my own.

As outlined by Dr. Beard, projections conducted eight to ten years ago, based on the age and numbers of the veteran population, make it quite evident that the last twenty years of this century will see a tripling in the number of veterans aged 65 and older. Furthermore, since the number of young people serving in the armed forces since World War II is approximately equal to the number that served during World War II, this preponderance of elderly veterans will continue well into the twenty-first century.

In 1973, it became obvious to Dr. Paul Haber, Director of Extended Care for the Veterans Administration, that it was time to attract good people to the field of geriatric medicine if the VA was to be responsible in its efforts to care for these older persons. The way to do it, Dr. Haber concluded, was through an approach that the Veterans Administration had found successful in other areas of medicine—through stressing education and research and linking these to clinical care under the same roof.

To apply these principles to a difficult area, such as geriatric medicine, is not easy and, in Dr. Haber's view, required a special approach. For this purpose, Dr. Haber and his colleagues proposed the creation of "centers of excellence"— the goal of which would be to "achieve professional legitimacy by attracting outstanding professionals to teach and conduct research in aging in a clinical context and, as a result, to have a positive impact on the care of the older veteran" [1]. In defining the broad outlines of this proposal, Dr. Haber specified that these centers should have strong affiliations with medical schools; their research programs should contain a mix of biomedical and psychosocial research; they should serve as regional educational centers in the area of geriatrics; and they should provide a model of geriatric practice for other hospitals to emulate.

Dr. Haber sought advice from members of the VA community who had demonstrated leadership in the field of geriatric medicine and long-term care concerning the specific design to be employed. Their advice was that the research should relate both to basic and clinical levels, that it should stress the aging focus, and that specific awards for research support should be made on the basis of peer review. The educational components should stress transmission of knowledge, acquisition of skills, and the development of attitudes, and should encompass preprofessional as well as graduate and continuing education. The clinical component should include small inpatient demonstration units with ambulatory care and consultative services added.

The concept included a specific provision that, in addition to assuming personal responsibility for a small inpatient service (specifically designed for special study and to serve as an evaluation center and educational focus), the director of these programs should also be placed in charge of *all* geriatric clinical functions at the medical center. This provision insured that the individual components already in place at the institution and necessary for comprehensive ongoing care would be coordinated into a single multilevel and multifaceted system. The broad mandate assigned to these centers was reflected in their name "Geriatric Research, Education, and Clinical Centers (GRECCs).

Development of fiscal authorization for this program was achieved in 1975. Seven centers were identified that seemed to contain potential for leadership in this field. These include the following: Bay Pines, Bedford/Boston OPD (where the Normative Aging Study had been in place for some years), Little Rock, Palo Alto, Seattle/American Lake, Sepulvada, and Wadsworth. A Request for Proposal was circulated. St. Louis was added and Minneapolis replaced Bay Pines, leaving eight centers in all. I am told that core funding is approximately 250 thousand dollars per center.

Clearly these centers provide a priceless asset to the university with which they are affiliated. I have had the privilege of visiting several of them. Two aspects of the program are immediately apparent. First is the number of independent, though related, teacher-investigators concerned with various aspects of aging, for which this program provides vital support—chiefly, I gather, in the form of professional salaries. This is in sharp contrast to VA Medical Centers that do not have this form of support, in which fully salaried physicians, interested in geriatrics and long-term care, are expected to devote their major energies to direct patient care. Second, as a result of the provision that the director of the

GRECC also serves as coordinator or director of *all* medical services within the Medical Center which relate to long-term care of older persons, those centers that are fortunate enough to receive GRECC support are able to develop and maintain a coordinated multilevel care system for older veterans in which all of the individual components work together smoothly within a single organized structure.

This is in contrast to most medical centers, as exemplified by our own, where ambulatory care and hospital-based home-care units relate administratively to the Associate Chief of Staff for Ambulatory Care; inpatient services relate to the Chief of Medicine and Chief of Staff; and the responsibility for recruitment, placement, and supervision of each professional group (physician, nurse, social worker, and so on) is specifically vested in the Office of the Director for that professional component. This type of administrative fragmentation is clearly inconsistent with the fundamental principles of interdisciplinary team care, which the VA stresses in other contexts. As a result, the potential for utilizing the dollars that are already invested in individual aspects of care for older persons, in the development of demonstration and teaching programs, and in comprehensive care is severely limited.

To what extent the medical profession should assume broad responsibility for social as well as health-related aspects of support to older persons is still a very important and debatable issue. One view has been expressed thus: "Social problems are increasingly being defined as medical conditions and health professionals, especially physicians, are being asked to solve problems for which they have no special knowledge or training" [2].

Dr. Haber's perspective on this point is illustrated by the following statement: "Many of the societal problems of the aged—housing, heating, feeding, and recreation—are being abrogated by society and laid on medicine's examining table. It is important to determine the confines of the broad term 'care'."

This issue remains an important one, with strong implications for the role that medicine will play in the area of aging. Some will express the view that it is hard enough for physicians to understand medicine and its fundamental disciplines of biology and psychology, without expecting them to understand and play a role in society's problems. Others will point out that, by confining the area of interest and responsibility of physicians, one limits them to the role of technicians. Some feel that this fosters an approach that already exists in some state mental hospitals, in which social scientists make all important administrative and policy decisions, and the role of physicians is limited to giving advice (when asked) and signing reports. One thing seems clear—if physicians are to play a role solving the broad issues facing society and the health-care system, physicians need to be more familiar with that system and with the disciplines required to understand it.

As I read over summaries of the deliberations that have taken place within the Division of Long-Term Care over the past eight years, I believe that Dr.

Haber, Dr. Goldman, and their colleagues have shared this view. Their concerns are reflected in the guidelines for the next two programs that I would like to describe.

The first is the Geriatric Physician Fellowship Program. For reasons that are not entirely evident in the material I have reviewed, the Central Office decided that establishment of GRECCs was not the only mechanism they would initiate in the development of educational programs in geriatrics and gerontology. In 1977/1978 the administration announced its intent to establish Geriatric Physician Fellowship Programs. These Programs would not be limited to GRECCs, but would be extended to other hospitals that indicated a commitment to medical education and to continuing care. The goals of this program, outlined in the Request for Proposal, are as follows: 1) to prepare physicians, board certified or eligible in internal medicine (including possibly its specialties), family medicine, or psychiatry for clinical excellence in geriatrics/gerontology; 2) to equip these individuals to function as clinicians, teachers and coordinators in inpatient and ambulatory care settings; and 3) to provide national leadership in geriatric education in VA facilities and affiliated medical schools. Fellowships, which extend over a two-year period, are funded at the level of "regular" VA physicians, commensurate with the individual's experience and qualifications. Emphasis is placed on multidisciplinary training in medicine (specifically long-term care), with linkages to physical medicine and rehabilitation, psychiatry, and other disciplines, such as social work and nursing.

The program incorporates a "systems approach" to program development and evaluation, including a somewhat controversial device known as a "learning contract," which is developed for each fellow after discussion between the applicant and program director, and with specific approval by the VA Central Office. Research activities are not stressed and, to the regret of some, are specifically minimized as part of this fellowship program, but are available, following competitive application, during a third year of support. The fellowships include a three-month experience in a European geriatric center.

Following submission of competitive applications, five centers were funded during the fiscal year 1978 and five additional programs were awarded during the following year. Each center is authorized to nominate two candidates for appointment each year. The VA centers which have been designated as sites of Geriatric Physician Fellowships are Bedford, Buffalo, Durham, Gainesville, Lexington, Little Rock, Madison, Palo Alto, Philadelphia, Portland, Sepulvada, and Wadsworth.

The success of this program has been gratifying to everyone involved. I am told that each of the fellows who will be completing their training in June 1980 have received an average of ten offers of positions in the field of geriatric medicine!

The final program I would like to describe is the Geriatric Interdisciplinary Team Training Program. The goals of this program, as stated in the Request for Proposal are threefold:

1. To foster the team approach to the care of the elderly.
2. To encourage affiliation with health profession schools in addition to medicine.
3. To translate what exists "or should exist" in the delivery system into the educational system.

Thus, this program reflects quite directly the concern about the system of care to which I have alluded earlier.

The goals of this program, as described in the background material, involve the establishment of interdisciplinary training models for health profession students and practitioners in clinical settings and the introduction of structured didactic and clinical interdisciplinary learning experiences. The objectives stress that the intent of the program is not only to foster an interface among professions but to insure that this interface is developed in such a way that it will reflect and teach group process skills. It has not been easy for a physician, such as myself, to understand what is meant by group process skills. One must understand activities, such as group decision-making process, verbal and nonverbal communication, identification of different leadership styles, and identification and resolution of interpersonal conflicts. More difficult, one must learn not only how to do these things but also how to teach them. The Request for Proposal concludes with the statement that "A collaborative team approach is more efficient, more effective, and more humane."

We have, with some difficulty, developed two successive applications for this program. The first was pronounced a disaster. We have not yet heard the results of our second application. We have learned at least *something* about group process skills in the preparation of these applications and are eager to give this approach an honest try. A review of the literature has, however, failed to provide documentation that this particular approach, as applied to long-term care of patients, is more efficient or more effective than traditional patterns of collaboration. These are difficult points to evaluate. If we do receive this award, we are determined to try to study this point through use of a matched controlled population.

In summary, therefore, the VA system provides unique assets in the development of an academic program in geriatric medicine. The leaders of the VA medical system have been among the first in this country to identify the provision of care to the elderly as an area of national need.

The system does have certain limitations, of course. The fact that most veterans are men while the preponderance of very old individuals are women is obvious. So, too is the fact that the patterns of referral, decision making, and funding inherent in the VA system are not representative of the American health-care system as a whole. One detects ambivalence among policy makers concerning the extent to which the benefits of this system should be provided to *all* veterans as opposed to those with service-connected disabilities. One inevitably wonders about the future of the VA system in a framework in which increasingly all care for older persons is being provided by some form of third-party mechanism, which is available to veterans as it is to others.

A bit more puzzling is the extent to which the administrative structure, which I gather is characteristic of most VA Medical Centers, divides the elements of care among different centers of responsibility, thus inhibiting the extent of coordination and integration that might otherwise be present.

When the VA system initiated these programs, few medical schools contained divisions or programs in geriatric medicine. Those who did were in a position to develop strong applications for GRECCs—applications that were strengthened by the fact, not unique to this particular situation, that staff members in these centers had participated in the development of the program design. Now a number of other medical schools are waiting in line. We have found that we must become expert in the *modus operandi* and goals of a variety of agencies. These include the National Institute on Aging (geriatric medicine academic awards); the Administration on Aging (long-term-care gerontology centers and fellowship programs); the Bureau of Health Manpower (curriculum development grants); the Johnson Foundation (community-based demonstration programs for support to the frail elderly); area and state Agencies on Aging, which play a vital role in "channeling grants"; and a variety of private foundations. The result is that faculty members, many of them full-time or part-time VA employees, are finding a need to spend large segments of time in "grantsmanship."

The key role played by the VA system is illustrated by the fact that, in the recent tour of geriatric facilities in Britain, Norway and Sweden, sponsored by the Administration on Aging for the recipients of demonstration grants for long-term-care centers, 66% of the physician-participants were based primarily in the VA system.

The Veterans Administration is emerging at the center of the arena in a national effort to provide better medical care and social support for our older citizens. The enfolding drama will be an interesting one to watch and to participate in.

References

1. "Background and Early History of the GRECC's" and other statements by Dr. Paul Haber, kindly provided by the VA Central Office, Washington, D.C.

2. Zola, I.K. In the name of health and illness: On socio-political consequences of medical influence. *Social Science and Medicine* 9:83, 1975.

12 Multiple Clinical Facilities in Geriatric Training with Emphasis on the Use of Community Service Agencies and a Role-Model Geriatrician—The Experience at Upstate Medical Center of New York— Binghamton Clinical Campus

Frank R. Brand, M.D.
Lawrence T. Tremonti, M.D.

The Binghamton Clinical Campus, as a community-based program in clinical medical education, was developed to allow for a significant and cost-effective expansion in the number of students receiving medical degrees and to provide for innovative medical education programs emphasizing primary care in all of its health care, prevention, and maintenance facts.

In 1975, the Board of Trustees of the State University of New York authorized Upstate Medical Center (UMC) and SUNY-Binghamton to proceed with the development of a community-based program in medical education. The Binghamton Clinical Campus was established as a unique partner of a traditional medical school with a geographically distant university center.

The Clinical Campus is designed to move medical education outside of the medical school tertiary-care hospital into community facilities, and in so doing to influence the geographic distribution of physician services, as well as choice of specialty. Specifically, the Clinical Campus has as a fundamental purpose the provision of clinical medical education for undergraduates, with special emphasis on the training aspects of primary care. A secondary goal is to build a functional system of medical education by utilizing the already-constructed medical care facilities of the NY-Penn HSA area, and, in the process, to improve the quality and quantity of care.

Facilities of the Clinical Campus are located on the Binghamton Campus of the State University of New York. The student body is comprised of approximately 25% of the third- and fourth-year classes from Upstate Medical Center in Syracuse. The students, who elect to join the Clinical Campus, move seventy-five miles south from Syracuse to Binghamton at the completion of their second year of medical school.

In developing the Clinical Campus curriculum, an epoch approach to life stages was utilized as it best addressed the goals of the Clinical Campus and fostered interdisciplinary relationships. This process resulted in a number of innovative programs, including a longitudinal continuity of care program designed to integrate the study of social, behavioral, and management sciences whose focus is on primary care. Another innovation, and the subject of this project, is the geriatrics/gerontology program.

The Clinical Campus effort generated a strong commitment to geriatric medicine as a significant and integral part of the school curriculum. A geriatric advisory committee and faculty had the unique opportunity to reflect on the best use of an allocated amount of student time in achieving the program objectives rather than spending energy contesting with stronger established departments for any student exposure at all. The result of these deliberations and subsequent experience with the established clinical facilities are the basis of this discussion.

There are four major aspects of the Clinical Campus geriatric program:

1. A required two-week geriatric clerkship
2. Six afternoon public health seminars
3. Weekly primary-care office experience
4. Fourth year electives

During our first year of operation, we concentrated on the required two-week clerkship. Although a two-week period of time to cover objectives in geriatric medicine may be in conflict with the time course approach to the geriatric patient, it is unlikely that any geriatric program will get a much greater segment of required student exposure, given the multiple forces hearing on curriculum time allocation.

The geriatric program committee, whose responsibility was to design and implement this effort, is composed of three part-time individuals including a physician educator, a health educator, and a social worker with strong counseling and academic background. Several decisions made during the planning phase of the geriatric clerkship have held up well during this first teaching year. Two important principles of adult continuing education generated over the last ten years were utilized: the need to allow choice in education procedure and the need of the adult to utilize past and recent experience during the educational experience. A third principle used was that of developing *both* physician and nonphysician preceptors. This was not a principle of adult education per se, but reflected our concerns about the need for the primary-care physician to relate effectively with a variety of resource persons during the course of education.

We also felt that there are phases of geriatric life, each of which requires special skills and knowledge by the practicing primary-care physician. These phases of geriatric life, which we have identified for curriculum and resource development, include: 1) the ambulatory well geriatric individual; 2) those dependent on community services; and 3) those geriatric individuals living in long-term-care institutions. The clinical facilities were identified to provide exposure and development of competence in each of these phases of geriatric life. These have been given equal weight in our effort because of the demands of each on the health-care system.

A brief enumeration of the special skills and knowledge necessary to deal with each of these patient groups will illustrate a spectrum of educational objectives. The needs of the ambulatory patient for preventive care, awareness by the physician of health predictors, and the need for health maintenance counseling is contrasted with the long-term-care skills of evaluation of debilitated patients, understanding of levels of care and commitment to the team approach to patient management. Interspersed between these two is the patient requiring support services and a primary-care physician knowledgeable about rehabilitation principles, specific services in a given community, and communication linkages with widely scattered health-service professionals.

When balancing the numbers of educational objectives with the time available in a two-week clerkship, we became committed to the strategy of a student focusing on one of the phases of geriatric life in order to avoid fragmentation of his experience. The clinical facilities that were chosen to develop the skills necessary in a given phase of geriatric life were community agencies, rehabilitation services, and long-term care.

The principles of adult education clearly identify the need of the adult student to exercise choice in his area of endeavor and to share his knowledge and expertise with a peer group. Some of our students brought significant prior knowledge to the clerkship from their past employment experience.

We decided to allow the student a choice in clinical facilities that addressed his own educational needs and interest, but we then had to develop a vehicle whereby the student group could share their experience and knowledge. Figure 12-1 depicts our educational strategy for the two-week clerkship. It shows an introductory morning emphasizing the goals of the program and the objectives of the clinical facilities. Two weeks earlier, the student had chosen the facility that best met his educational objectives. The illustration shows an unexpected fourth track labeled Role Model Geriatrician, which evolved from the long-term-care track and will be explained later in detail. Following two weeks of experience in the clinical facilities, the students met in a seminar session to share their experience with the different delivery models. Interspersed throughout the clerkships are reading assignments and afternoon small group seminars involving attitudes, case discussions, and counseling.

As other chapters discuss in depth geriatric teaching in long-term-care facilities and the general hospital and outreach medical services, the rehabilitation and long-term-care clerkships will receive only passing comment. The two experiences that we would like to discuss more completely are the community service experience and the role model geriatrician.

The community service preceptorship is available through the Office for

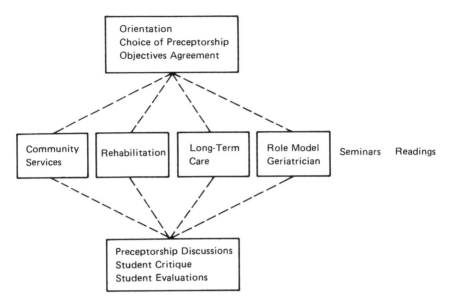

Figure 12-1. Geriatric Curriculum Strategy for Two-Week Clerkship.

Aging and the Public Health Department. As with most community facilities, their great strengths are their experience with the problems of the elderly and their enthusiasm to share that knowledge. Their most prominent weakness is a lack of credentials in the traditional mode and experience in education. It was fortunate that each member of our geriatric faculty has a significant background in various aspects of education. The objectives of the preceptorship are to:

1. Create an awareness of the goals of Area Agencies on Aging
2. Instill knowledge of the range of services available
3. Develop a positive view toward the elderly as a vital, active, and capable population
4. Effectively demonstrate the importance of economic, emotional, and social factors that affect wellness or illness of the geriatric population, so that such will be an integral part of the data gathering
5. Teach how best to make client referrals to appropriate community agencies.

Some of the specific activities of the community service preceptorship deserve further discussion. These are described in order according to their evaluation by the still-limited number of students who have completed the program. The students felt that the most important activity to them as future primary-care physicians was the opportunity to participate in client counseling sessions concerning nutrition, finances, and mental health. Clients were referred to the counselors by public health nurses in the field, workers at adult activity centers, or informed primary-care physicians. Counseling services are available within the facilities of the Office for Aging and are conducted by nutritionists, social workers, or psychologists. Another student activity is to make home visits with public health nurses. This was viewed by the students as valuable and is well discussed elsewhere. The Office for Aging in our community schedules team conferences for clients who require coordination of multiple community facilities. The students felt that this activity was worthwhile, but they tended to be observers rather than actually involved in the decisions for these particular clients. Students also visited adult activity centers of the Office for Aging. This gave them the opportunity to see the healthy elderly in social relationships. The students felt that this activity did not provide enough value to them as future primary-care physicians when balanced against the time allotment for activity centers in the preceptorship.

The community service preceptorship exposes the student to the vital elderly receiving services necessary to maintain that condition. The community agency contains numerous opportunities for the student to explore the important issues that affect this age group, such as the availability of physician care and the implications of fixed income in an inflationary economy and social isolation. Within these agencies there are potentially unique and rich experiences with agency administrators, nurses in an outreach setting, nutritionists, and other providers. The student has the opportunity to develop functioning educational relationships with excellent nonphysician preceptors.

On the other hand, because of the numerous activities of these agencies, it is possible for the students to fall into a pattern of poorly interrelating visits to various delivery settings. In addition, the student may have a sense of being an observer only, unless a specific set of tasks is given. The health professionals in this area must be given adequate educational support by the medical education system in establishing objectives and procedures for each student. Also, the student should be given specific tasks to lend structure to his experience and to facilitate dealing with the elderly. We have found information gathering in areas of client nutrition, economic pressures and physician utilization to be valuable educational experiences. Care has been taken to have the students integrate this information to data gathering in health delivery of the primary-care physician.

The primary care geriatrician is able to expose the student to the three types of patients previously noted: the ambulatory individual, the person requiring community services, and the institutionalized patient. This faculty person has the unique opportunity to assign the student to patients who are about to make the transition from the hospital to other environments. The hospitalized patients who are awaiting placement demand of the student a concern for family interplay, proper choice of supportive outpatient care or institutional care, and an understanding of the financial impact of supportive care for the elderly.

The geriatrician is rare in middle-sized New York cities. At least in our experience, the ideal preceptor is the medical director who maintains an active primary-care practice. We have found only two such individuals in our own setting who have expressed a willingness to teach.

The objectives of this preceptorship are:

1. To have the students demonstrate competence in dealing with well ambulatory elderly. This is to include adequate communication with the patient, concerns for health maintenance, and awareness of the social and economic factors that come into play with elderly patients.
2. To have the students be capable of evaluation of patients in transition from acute hospital into chronic-care institutions or community support structures.
3. To have the student be aware of the principles of the team approach to meet the needs of the elderly in long-term settings.

The specific activities that were reviewed by the students for the role model geriatrician preceptorship included formal discussion, patient workups and community agency visits. Drawing again upon our limited experience, students felt that the most valuable aspect of this preceptorship was the opportunity to discuss the philosophy of care of geriatric patients with a resource person whom they respect. Another aspect of the preceptorship is the workup of two patients in each of the epochs of geriatric life. That is, the student had the opportunity to evaluate two patients who were well and ambulatory, two in a community hospital in transition, and two patients in a long-term-care setting. The evaluation of these patients included not only carrying out a history and physical examination, but planning for continuing management. The students felt this activity was very worthwhile, especially the opportunity to think about and present a plan for the continuing welfare of the patient. The geriatrician also arranged for some visits by the student to the community agencies, but this experience was brief and somewhat fragmented. The students felt they were able to gain this type of information from their seminars with other students specifically assigned to community agencies.

This preceptorship has the very marked advantage of exposing the student to the major epochs of geriatric life in an orderly and well-supervised fashion. The student is also provided with a role model for geriatric management. This preceptorship also offers the opportunity for significant amounts of informational interplay between student and preceptor focusing on the major social and economic problems of the elderly. It also has the potential of stimulating cooperative research with the preceptors involving aspects of either institutional care or management of the healthy elderly adult.

On the other hand, this preceptorship has the tendency to reinforce the "totally physician directed" health-care system. This is in conflict with one of the objectives of the geriatric clerkship, which is to expose the student to non-physician educators. The other difficulty with this preceptorship is that role model geriatricians are rare and cannot serve as preceptors for significant numbers of medical students. It does, however, serve the purpose of establishing a model for demonstrating the spectrum of geriatric care. This can be used in research and development of other more-available clinical facilities.

Student response to the program has been quite favorable, although it must be remembered that this is a selected population of medical students. These students have elected to come to the Clinical Campus knowing that the emphasis would be on training of the primary-care physician.

The role model geriatrician, as might be expected, consistently received the highest ratings from the students. The students that selected the community service preceptorship felt that they had greatly expanded their potential as primary-care physicians. This is important with respect to our educational objectives because the preceptors in this experience are largely nonphysicians.

The rehabilitation and chronic-care experiences received above-average ratings, although generally the students were concerned about the inability to follow rehabilitation patients throughout the patient's experience because of the two-week limitation of the rotation.

Our experience with multiple clinic facilities in a geriatric clerkship have been described. The use of principles of adult continuing education are valuable in broadening the experience of the entire student group on a particular rotation. Four educational tracks were devised for student choice. Detailed evaluation of two of them, community agency experience and exposure to a role model geriatrician, reveal their strengths and weaknesses in the training of medical students self-directed to primary care.

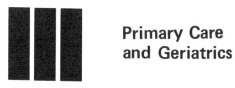

Primary Care
and Geriatrics

13 Introduction

Gerald R. Gehringer, M.D.

This section, dealing with the relationship of geriatrics to the delivery of primary care, attempts to identify the basic needs of the aging person. Once detailed, the section defines objectives and their implementation in the education of the primary-care physician.

The chapters by James Conover and Ethel Shanas, Ph.D. address the medical and social needs of the older individual that must be considered by the primary-care physician. M. William Voss, M.D. then presents the viewpoint of one such doctor.

Opportunities to meet the needs of the geriatric patient in the training programs of both family practitioners and internists are then presented by Richard Ham, M.D., assisted by Michelle L. Marcy, M.S. and Marcia Smith, Ph.D. They comment on the design of modules and the use of journals and texts for students and practitioners alike. The need for teaching geriatrics in a variety of settings, at all levels of medical education, and for all types of health care professionals is emphasized.

Evan Calkins, addresses the establishment of a geriatric unit in academic medicine from the viewpoint of an internist. He adds to the "three-legged stool" of academia (care, research, and teaching) a fourth leg of community involvement. He also emphasizes the necessity of support from the institution and other departments.

Looking to models where both primary care and geriatrics are well developed, David Carboni, Ph.D. presents an analysis of geriatrics in the United Kingdom. Since programs in primary care utilize the ambulatory setting to such a great degree, Jon D. Calvert, M.D., Ph.D. and Hugo K. Koch, M.H.A. detail the demographic data, which forms the basis for the need for primary care training in geriatrics. Their chapter concludes by listing six areas for special consideration when developing the ambulatory component of a geriatric curriculum.

Joseph Holtzman, Ph.D. concludes this section by highlighting the need for a research base for geriatrics even within the primary-care setting. Further, he proposes in broad terms a research agenda.

14 Primary Care: What the Elderly Want

James F. Conover

As a so-called "senior citizen" in a period of life described as the "golden years," I am at risk of being placed in a CAT scanner to discover what internal clock keeps me ticking. Furthermore, it must not be presumed that I speak for the more than 24 million Americans who have managed somehow to live 65 or more years. I assure you I am not presumptuous enough to think I can do so! Older people are as diverse in viewpoints and attitudes and as engaging or abrasive in manner as any other age group in this nation. What I have to present will therefore necessarily be subjective, although I shall try to express what I perceive to be some of the views of other older Americans.

I asked a friend of mine who is hale and hearty at the relatively tender age of 75 for his thoughts about doctors. "Obviously, we couldn't get along without doctors," he said, "and I rank them very high among our professional people. But I can also tell you, one of my main aims in life is to call on them as seldom as possible."

All of us recognize that age is a relative thing, depending to a large extent upon one's attitude toward life. Satchel Paige, the baseball pitcher who pitched 64 consecutive scoreless innings when he was more than 40 years old, once asked: "How old would you *be* if you didn't know how old you *was*?" When Coco Chanel of French-perfume fame was asked her age by a newspaper reporter, she is reputed to have answered: "My age varies according to the day and the people I happen to be with. When I'm bored, I feel very old, and since I'm extremely bored with you, I'm going to feel like a thousand years old if you don't get the hell out of here."

As a layman and as a beneficiary of the developments of geriatric education, I would like to address what I find encouraging in recent developments in geriatric medicine and I would also like to suggest a few ways in which geriatric medicine might be strengthened and the doctor-patient relationship improved.

On the positive side, we have seen a burgeoning of interest in research and medical education designed specifically to keep older people in better physical and mental health. This has been reflected in the outpouring of books and articles dealing with the social, economic, psychological, and physical aspects of aging. It is reflected in the heightened awareness by state and federal legislators of the fact that they have an increasing number of older constituents whose needs must be taken into account. It is reflected in the recognition by medical schools and teaching hospitals that those who are training to be doctors, nurses, and medical technicians need broader exposure to the many facets of geriatric medicine. It is reflected in the establishment of the National Institute of Aging, under the vigorous leadership of Dr. Robert N. Butler. And it is reflected in the increasing efforts to seek new directions in health care for older Americans. So we have many reasons to be encouraged by recent trends in geriatric education and in the practice of geriatric medicine, but I have the temerity to suggest—from a layman's viewpoint—that there are a number of areas where improvements could be made.

There is a need for primary-care physicians to have better knowledge of the symptomatic effects of various illnesses in older people so that correct diagnoses can be made. I understand from no less an authority than Dr. Butler that the reactions of older people to certain illnesses may differ from those of younger people.

There is also a need for someone to marshal all available social and home health-care services to help the older patient. A conference on geriatric medicine in 1979 sponsored by the National Retired Teachers Association and the American Association of Retired Persons made special note of this issue. Whether the primary-care physician should serve as captain of the health-care team arranging these services, or whether a nurse, social service worker, or other professional should function in this essential but time-consuming role can be debated.

There is a need for primary-care physicians to have a greater appreciation of, and commitment to, preventive health measures. Physicians who are paid salaries by health maintenance organizations likely have a greater incentive than physicians in private practice to help their patients avoid expensive care in hospitals and nursing homes. I am convinced that we can do much more, for example, through proper diet, adequate exercise, and control of certain diseases to help older Americans maintain reasonably good health and avoid serious illness.

Only about 5% of older Americans are residents of nursing homes and other long-term-care institutions at any time, but these debilitated and chronically ill persons are the ones who require genuinely sympathetic and intelligent care. What is the role of the primary-care physician toward the patients he may have treated for years but who are consigned to nursing homes? Does the doctor's responsibility end, or should the doctor continue to check on the mental and physical health of these individuals.

There is a need for hospice-type services to help terminally ill patients accept the eventuality of death as gracefully, courageously, and painlessly as possible. I am confident we could learn from other nations that have considered the need to ease the physical and spiritual trauma of dying. For example, it seems foolish to be reluctant to prescribe sufficient medication to control the pain of the terminally ill patient because of the drug's addictive properties. There is no reason to allow a dying patient cycles of pain interspersed with relief when adequate quantities of analgesics provide a relatively painfree period prior to death.

In addition to our interest in the quality of clinical medicine, the 12.5 million members of the two associations I represent are seriously concerned about the soaring cost of hospital and medical care. Health-care costs, which have greatly outpaced the inflation rate and most other items in the consumer price index, have been doubling about every five years. It is ironic that people who are 65 years of age or older are now paying more for health care out of their pocket than this segment of the population did prior to 1965, the first year of Medicare, when third-party payer covered approximately 80% of medical and hospital costs of older citizens. Today it covers only about 74% of hospital costs and 55% of physicians' fees. Older Americans as a group have smaller incomes than younger persons, and many find it difficult or impossible to pay for adequate health care. In 1979 the Carter Administration urged Congress to impose mandatory cost controls on hospitals so as to limit their increase in expenses to approximately 11.6% a year. The associations I represent strongly supported this legislation. However, only a bill urging voluntary controls was passed.

Our associations have also supported passage of the Health Care for All Americans Act, which would provide quality health care for all Americans, regardless of age or income. Under this act, health-care expenditures would be permitted to rise only at the rate of growth of our gross national product. Every year a national health insurance board would set budgets for state and national health-care costs. Within each state, a planning board would set budgets for hospitals, and the consumers of health care would negotiate fee schedules with physicians and other providers.

We are convinced that ultimately we shall follow the example of virtually all industrialized nations of the world and enact a comprehensive, cost-conscious, national health insurance plan. We contend that good health care is a basic right for all of our people, young or old, rich or poor.

Our associations can claim credit for a vigorous national campaign that has induced 46 states to pass legislation either permitting or requiring the use of lower-priced generic drugs in place of equivalent higher-priced brand name drugs. This legislation is now saving millions of dollars each year for persons, many of whom are elderly, who need prescription drugs.

The need is clear for a continuation and expansion of basic research to shed new light on the mental and physical health problems of older Americans. The support of our associations for such grants is wholehearted. Although a major proportion of the funds required for research must come from government, additional help is needed from private foundations. Our members contributed more than two million dollars to establish the Ethel Percy Andrus Gerontology Center at the University of Southern California as a memorial to the remarkable woman who founded our two associations. Furthermore, in 1973, the NRTA-AARP Andrus Foundation was organized to serve as a continuing medium for the support of research in aging and human development. The Andrus Foundation has funded 91 research grants through 44 colleges and universities, at a cost of more than 2 million dollars.

It is not our objective to prolong the normal life span, but rather to improve the quality of life in the later years. Hence, we would like to see more investigation into the chronic debilitating illnesses, such as arthritis and senile dementia. If we could improve the condition of even 5% of those thought to be suffering from senile dementia, the effort would be eminently worthwhile.

We are encouraged that so many of the nation's 120 medical schools are now giving their students some exposure to geriatric medicine. At the same time, our associations do not advocate that geriatric medicine be turned into a specialty. Most of us have developed a special personal relationship with our primary-care physician, and we do not wish to change doctors just because we are getting old. Moreover, if geriatrics were a full specialty, wouldn't that tend to absolve primary-care physicians of their responsibility to provide intelligent treatment to their older patients?

We think the best solution is to interweave instruction in geriatric medicine throughout the medical school curriculum. We recommend that a geriatric curriculum be developed in all four years of medical school and in the postgraduate years and include exposure to older persons who reside in long-term-care institutions.

I am grateful to have an opportunity to present a layperson's point of view. Through patient and persistent efforts to improve geriatric education, new directions in health care can be made that will benefit future generations of older Americans.

15 The Health Needs of the Elderly: A Social-Medical Problem

Ethel Shanas, Ph.D.

Meeting the health needs of the elderly in the United States, as in other countries, is a social-medical problem. This social-medical problem cannot be solved solely by the expenditure of more funds for care of the elderly or by the training of more physicians, or by exhortations to members of families to face up to their responsibilities to their kith and kin. Proper health care of the elderly requires all of this as well as a recognition of the special problems that confront the elderly and an attempt at imaginative and nontraditional solutions. A World Health Organization report has summarized the situation very well: ". . . . good intentions will be harmful rather than helpful, particularly if attempts are made to solve non-medical problems by medical methods and techniques. Medical factors can often be overemphasized because individuals often mention medical problems first, this being easier and more acceptable. There may, however, be underlying social and economic problems of greater importance" [1].

To understand why the health needs of the elderly are a social-medical problem we need to consider the numbers of older people and some of their demographic characteristics, the health of the elderly, and the kinds of health services required by older people.

The Elderly Population

When is a person old? There is no simple answer to this question. All the research evidence available shows that people grow old at different rates. One person may be physically old at 60 while another is young at 75. There is a need for a definition of old age based on function rather than on the calendar. The components of what such a definition should be are as yet undetermined [2].

In this country, we usually describe as old those persons aged 65 and over. Such persons are sometimes euphemistically called "golden agers" or "senior citizens." In this chapter they are identified as "older people" or the "elderly." Current estimates are that there are now about 24.5 million persons aged 65 and over in the United States who comprise about 11% of the American population. Of these 24.5 million persons, about 5 million are aged 80 and over and about 2 million are over the age of 85 [3]. It is those old people aged 80 plus that particularly present the physician with social as well as medical problems.

Living to 80 is living to a "good age," beyond the Biblical threescore and ten. Men who live to be 80 on the average can expect to live 6.9 more years; women 9 more years. Men who live to be 85 can expect on the average to live 5.5 more years; women 6.9 more years [4]. Eighty years of age, then, is for many not an end point but simply one more birthday on the way to being 90 or older. Unfortunately, as people live longer they are more likely to be sick.

The usual patient aged 80 and over is a woman. She is a widow with a limited income [5], and she has a variety of physical complaints (an average of four), not all of which can be cured or even alleviated.

Despite popular belief, most people aged 80 and over are not in institutions. At any one time, one of every eight will be in an institution, primarily in a nursing home [6]. Based on discharge data that indicate that nursing home beds turn over once in the course of a year, one can estimate that about one of every four persons now aged 80 and over will spend some time in a nursing home in any one year [7,8]. Some persons die in the nursing home, others are discharged from the nursing home to another health facility and die there, still others are discharged from the nursing home or health facility to a private or semiprivate residence where they continue to live for an undetermined period.

The Health of the Elderly

At this time, about 95% of all Americans aged 65 and over are living in the community, either with a spouse, with children, or on their own. Living alone is often a matter of choice for older people as it is for their adult grandchildren. Among older Americans in the community (according to a 1975 survey), one in every ten was bedfast and/or totally housebound. Thus, there were twice as many older Americans bedfast and housebound at home in 1975 as there were in institutions of all kinds. An additional one of every fourteen older persons could go outdoors only with difficulty. Thus about 2.7 million older persons in 1975 (about 17% of the population aged 65 and over) were bedfast, housebound, or otherwise limited in mobility and living at home. Of all persons over 65 living at home, about one of every four reported that at least one day was spent in bed because of illness during the year before the interview. About one person in every 100 (about 250,000 persons) reported that they had fallen during the previous week as the aftermath of a dizzy spell. Among those over 80, about one in every eight said they had fallen [9]. Despite these statistics, half of all old people, including half of those over 80, described their health as "good," and more than half said their health was better than the health of other people their age. However, one in every three older persons said that they had seen a doctor during the month before they were interviewed [9]. Some were undoubtedly acutely ill; however, most were chronically ill. Coping with the chronic illnesses of older patients is a challenge to the physician. The doctor can treat acute illness but often the symptoms of the chronically ill can only be alleviated.

Some years ago, Dr. Robert T. Monroe, a pioneer in the study of the diseases of the aged, said "if sickness is a pathologic state in some organ or tissue, then all old people are sick" [10]. The physician treating the elderly consciously or by default usually agrees with Dr. Monroe. On a practical level, a social definition of illness in the elderly has usually been accepted. As Dr. Monroe suggested, it is a degree of fitness rather than a degree of pathology that is the best measure of sickness or wellness among older people.

The Need for Care

The health care needs of older people vary. They change through time and are not met solely in the traditional settings of hospital, physician's office, and nursing home [11]. The hospital and the physician's office are appropriate settings for acute care or short-term care. The great need in care for the elderly, however, is long-term care. Because such needed care may differ from what is traditionally seen as health care, providers of health services may either be unaware of available services or inclined to exclude them from consideration when they plan the treatment of the older patient.

To begin with, the major resource in the care of the elderly is the family. Families are the primary caretakers of that one in ten among the elderly who is bedfast and housebound at home, and of that one in four who is ill enough to report spending a day in bed in a twelve-month period [9]. Families turn to institutions for the aged to care for their older relatives when all other resources are exhausted.

Long-term care for older people at home can be made possible by the provision of homemaker services. Such services can include help with housework, shopping, assistance with dressing and bathing, meal preparation, and so on. None of these services are strictly health services but they can be critical in determining whether an older person remains at home or enters an institution. Home health services, providing primarily nursing care but also meeting other medical and rehabilitative needs of the older patient, are also a necessary component of the long-term-care continuum. The payment schemes under which reimbursements are made for homemakers and home health services now in effect have resulted in these necessary programs being both fragmented and underutilized.

Adult day care and day hospital programs also provide services to the long-term-care patient. Adult day care provides health and social services to persons who can be transported between their homes and the care centers. Many of these centers focus primarily on the social needs of their clientele, while some provide physical, occupational, and other therapies on an ambulatory basis. The day hospital programs, in contrast to adult day care, usually concentrate on the rehabilitation of persons who have had strokes or serious physical injuries. Because of this emphasis day hospitals are usually associated with a health institution. Day hospitals have not been widely developed in the United States but are essential parts of the health system in many European countries, for example, Britain and Sweden [11,12].

Nursing homes are the most widely used component of long-term care for the elderly. In 1977, there were roughly 18,900 nursing homes in the United States, which provided 1,402,400 patient beds. There were 1,303,100 patients in nursing homes in late 1977 and 86% of them were aged 65 and over. The median age of residents in nursing homes was 81 years [13]. There seem to be two separate groups of persons who use nursing homes: those admitted for relatively short periods because recuperative care is needed, and "those admitted for relatively long periods of time because there is little chance of their chronic condition improving" [7]. Of all nursing home residents, 25% were dependent in all activities of daily living: mobility, bathing, dressing, using the toilet, continence, and eating.

Before suggesting admittance to a nursing home for an older patient, the physician should consider whether the nursing home really represents the best environment for that patient or whether some other care option should be investigated. It is the physician's responsibility to help both older people and their families consider the spectrum of services in long-term care.

New Approaches in Meeting the Health Needs of the Elderly

The numbers of older people and their survival to advanced ages has had a major influence on traditional approaches to meeting the health needs of the elderly. These new approaches involve the active enlistment of family care-givers, and they involve old people themselves. Health personnel are assuming new and different responsibilities. The physician with long-term-care patients must be willing to work closely with nursing personnel and physician's assistants so that they can assume major responsibility for day-to-day decision-making on patient care. A World Health Organization report states ". . . other health workers, including physicians, would only be involved (in the care of the patient) as a result of referral by the nurse" [14].

Wherever possible, every effort should be made to encourage home care of the long-term-care patient. This is what many patients and their families want. The delivery of such care involves social, emotional, and financial sacrifices by family members. Studies made in Ohio and North Carolina [15] indicate that families will assume the health care of elderly relatives, in addition to their parents and grandparents, if supportive services are made available to them. Actions speak louder than attitudes. At any one time, twice as many bedfast and housebound persons are taken care of in the community as in institutions of all kinds.

Finally, older people themselves are now assuming more responsibility for medical self-care, both as individuals and as members of self-help groups. Such medical self-care is not new. To quote from a National Institute of Health publication: "Patients with a chronic disease have been performing 'professional' tasks for years" [13]. The document, "A Guide to Medical Self-Care and Self-Help Groups for the Elderly," goes on to mention diabetics and persons with angina as persons who have been taking care of themselves, under physician directions, for many years. Older people are urged to follow good health practices and to learn how to make self-care judgements wisely. Further, older people are urged to participate in patient self-help groups, such as Reach for Recovery, Stroke Clubs, Arthritis Clubs and Emphysema Clubs, all of which teach techniques and skills that can ease day-to-day living [13].

The physician who is to treat the elderly patient faces new challenges. He or she must be prepared for changes in the roles of other health personnel; for the involvement of families; and for the extra time needed to listen to an older patient and to help the patient cope with a failing body. The patient, whether aged 65 or 90, just as the young adult, is something more than an ailing organ system or a disease.

References

1. World Health Organization, Regional Office for Europe. *Rehabilitation in Long-Term and Geriatric Care.* Copenhagen: World Health Organization, 1974.

2. Birren, J.E. and Renner, V.J. Research on the psychology of aging. Principles and experimentation. In J.E. Birren and K.W. Schaie (Eds.), *Handbook of the Psychology of Aging.* New York; Van Nostrand-Reinhold, 1977.

3. Siegel, J.S. *Demographic Aspects of Aging and the Older Population of the United States.* U.S. Bureau of the Census Current Population Reports. Series P-23, No. 59. Washington, D.C.: Government Printing Office, 1976.

4. U.S. Department of Health, Education, and Welfare. *Vital Statistics of the United States. Life Tables.* Vol. 2, Sec. 5. PHS Publication No. 80-1104. Hyattsville Maryland: National Center for Health Statistics, 1980.

5. Glick, P.C. The future marital status and living arrangements of the elderly. *The Gerontologist* 19(3):301, 1979.

6. U.S. Bureau of the Census. *Social and Economic Characteristics of the Older Population, 1978.* Current Population Reports. Series P-23, No. 85. Washington, D.C.: Government Printing Office, 1978.

7. U.S. Department of Health, Education and Welfare. *A Comparison of Nursing Residents and Discharges from the 1977 National Nursing Home Survey: United States.* Advance Data from Vital and Health Statistics of the National Center for Health Statistics. No. 29 (May 17). Hyattsville, Maryland: National Center for Health Statistics, 1978.

8. U.S. Department of Health, Education and Welfare, *The National*

Nursing Home Survey. Series 13, No. 43, (July). PHS Publication No. 79-1794. Hyattsville, Maryland: National Center for Health Statistics, 1979.

9. Shanas, E. National Survey of the Aged. A final report to the Administration on Aging, Project 90-A-369, HEW OHD, 1978.

10. Monroe, R.T. How well are older people? *J. Michigan State Med. Soc.* 59:748, 1960.

11. Weissert, W.G. Long-term care: An overview. In *Health United States.* PHS Publication No. 78-1232. Hyattsville, Maryland, U.S. Department of Health, Education, and Welfare, 1978.

12. Bozzetti, L.P. and Sherman, S. *The Aged in Sweden. I. the Country, its People and Institutions.* A Psychiatric Annals Reprint, New York: Insight Publishing Co., 1977.

13. U.S. Department of Health, Education and Welfare. *A Guide to Medical Self-Care and Self-Help Groups for the Elderly.* N.I.H. Publication No. 80-1687. Washington, D.C.: Government Printing Office, 1977.

14. Baker, D.E. The role of nursing in care of the elderly. In *World Health Organization, Regional Office for Europe, Nursing Aspects in the Care of the Elderly.* Report on a Working Group. Copenhagen: World Health Organization, 1977.

15. Sussman, M.B. et al. Social and Economic Supports and Family Environments for the Elderly. Administration on Aging Grant #90-A-316. Unpublished communication.

16 The Viewpoint of a Primary-Care Physician

M. William Voss, M.D.

A panel presentation and discussion recently outlined two special factors that have great importance if the medical needs of the elderly are to be met by primary-care doctors [1]. First, primary-care physicians must recognize that the older segment of the population is increasing. As noted, the contingent of the United States that is elderly has changed from 4% of the whole in the early 1900s to 10% in 1977 and may reach almost 20% by the year 2030 [2]. Translated into primary-care time, it is estimated that the component of total time devoted to the care of older Americans by the medical profession (currently 37%) will escalate to 75% in two generations.

Second, the medical profession has become increasingly subspecialized. This change has produced significant effects in types of care and their cost as well as widened the interpersonal distance between physician and patient. The average elderly person cannot, in many instances, traverse the health-care system alone and obtain acceptable medical care. The consequences of these two factors has made the problem of finding a primary-care physician the first need of the elderly patient.

The primary-care physician who has the responsibility for the management of an elderly person fulfills this responsibility with an approach that is global and unique. On the one hand, this relationship extends beyond specific medical needs to social, economic, spiritual and psychological areas. On the other hand, it is unique in that each patient is a very special individual, a composite of variables. Taken together, they can preclude that person from fitting well into protocols for purposes of diagnosis or therapy. In addition, many of the clinical skills applicable to the care of the elderly are different from those required for the care of a younger population.

The doctor delivering primary care often develops an extremely complex relationship with an elderly patient. For example, over the past decade the physician-elderly patient relationship has become increasingly legalistic. Strictly "medical codes" of behavior are less universely accepted and there is a need for both the physician and the patient to fully understand each other as they fulfill their roles in the "medical contract." Although this trend is seen at all points of contact between physician and patient and between all physicians and every patient of every age, this direction of medical care has special relevance to the primary-care physician and the elderly patient. Thus, patients' rights are often highlighted in discussions about nursing-home placement and the right to die.

Nonetheless, older people come to primary-care physicians mainly for medical care. Most (80%) of the elderly have some chronic medical condition [3]. The distribution of common complaints, with minor variations for ethnic, geographic, and occupational differences relate to the following systems: musculoskeletal (13%), skin (11%), gastrointestinal (10%), genitourinary (8.5%), vision and hearing (5%), and respiratory (5%). Fifteen percent of visits are prompted by the need for annual screening, and the remainder include appointments to manage complaints related to alcoholism, mood abnormalities (depression, agitation, and aggression), and mentation (memory loss, confusion, and personality change). Furthermore, the elderly often have multiple physical disorders that can be of unexpected urgency and diagnostic difficulty [4].

Although the majority of presenting conditions are physical, they are often associated with emotional reactions that require attention. Interwoven in many of these conditions are poverty, malnutrition, stress, and concerns about being the victims of crime [5]. The primary-care physician should take the lead in an interdisciplinary approach to meeting these complex needs.

Thus, the concept of primary care geriatric medicine includes aspects of "quality of life" and "degrees of wellness" as well as the more traditional concerns of diagnosis and treatment of disease. In providing continuity of care, the primary-care physician may be able to identify many aspects of preventive medicine that are important to the older patient as well.

The complex care of the elderly is intricately involved with family dynamics. Properly utilized, the family is the ideal and the strongest support system an elderly patient has. Social attitudes and emotional factors surrounding aging and death often deplete the energies of both patient and family. Through the primary-care physician, the family can be helped to fulfill its role in the care of its elders.

Finally, the elderly patient needs and requires assistance with what often appears to be an irrational health-benefits system. The primary-care physician can, as a patient advocate and health-care provider, advise, where necessary, and confront the system, where appropriate.

References

1. Guyther, R., Reichel, W., and Voss, M.W. The Family Physician in the Care of the Elderly, Past, Present, and Future. Panel Presentation and Discussion at the 1980 Annual Medical and Chirurgical Faculty of the State of Maryland Meeting.

2. Butler, R.N. The gray revolution and health—Coming of age. *Am. Pharm.* NS20(5):249, 1980.

3. Eckstein, D. Common complaints of the elderly. In W. Reichel (Ed.), *The Geriatric Patient.* New York: H.P. Publishing Co. Inc, 1978.

4. Wilson L.A., Lawson, I.R., and Brass, W. Multiple disorders of the elderly. A clinical and statistical study. *Lancet* 2:841, 1962.

5. Butler, R. Symposium on mental health and aging: Life cycle perspectives. *Geriatrics* 29:59, 1974.

17 Teaching Primary-Care Geriatrics

Richard J. Ham, M.D.
Michelle L. Marcy, M.S.
Marcia R. Smith, Ph.D.

It is clear that there are unmet health-care needs in the elderly population. We must, therefore, increase our efforts to establish and improve education in geriatrics at all levels of medical education, among health-care professionals and the general public.

The questions that we will address are:

1. What kind of educational experiences need to be provided?
2. Who should benefit from these educational experiences?
3. Who should provide them?

Primary care is that component of care that the elderly most lack in the United States today. In the development of the American medical system, acute care has been emphasized to the exclusion of chronic care, preventive care or the promotion of health. Whereas secondary or tertiary care are often excellent, access to such services is haphazard, sometimes resulting in either overtreatment or undertreatment.

Primary care has been defined as being characterized by accessibility, continuity, coordination, comprehensiveness, and accountability. These are all characteristics that anyone treating the elderly will understand as being important. Accessibility and accountability are particularly vital in those circumstances where confusion, fear, and financial barriers can prevent elderly patients from seeking health care and receiving appropriate follow-up attention. Continuity, coordination, and comprehensiveness are essential so that the person of first contact with the patient can intervene in the complex interplay of physical, psychological, and social factors in the treatment of illness in elderly people.

Skills needed to care for the elderly are not uniquely required by any one medical specialty. Indeed, every physician needs to be aware of the challenges and problems of caring for and communicating with the elderly. Even if the chosen specialty is pediatrics, the physician may have to relate to older relatives. Even if the physician is not going to engage in clinical work, there must be an appreciation of the importance of the relationship of aging to medical care if any effort is to have clinical significance and relevance. Thus, experiences in geriatrics must be a requirement for all medical students. Many schools are now attempting to fill the gaps described, for example, Southern Illinois University School of Medicine has a course of required experiences [1].

Too often, the medical student's sole exposure to elderly patients consists of acute-hospital experiences where older patients can easily be seen as time-consuming and unrewarding since they frequently are confused and unable to give a detailed history or even fully cooperate in the physical examination. When only hospitalized elderly patients are focused on, the rich and fascinating blend of psychosocial and medical problems can be perceived as a nuisance and a barrier to "proper" medical care. Thus, experiences for students must include exposure to elderly patients in the office, community, and home setting in order to encourage positive attitudes on the part of students. By seeing well elderly patients and those with medical problems who are coping in the community, the realistic possibility of a satisfactory outcome to acute or chronic illness in the elderly can be thoroughly appreciated. Thus, the increasing negativity toward the elderly that has been seen to occur during the process of medical education can be effectively countered [2,3].

How effective are geriatric programs in promoting medical students' positive attitudes toward elderly patients on the part of medical students? There have been a number of studies demonstrating that resident physicians have more negative attitudes toward the elderly than fourth-year students and practicing physicians have more negative attitudes still [4,5,6]. Therefore, student experiences must be carefully designed to engender understanding, empathy, and enthusiasm. It is not enough to offer didactic lectures or even the most sensitive small group discussions. Students need to have well-supervised clinical responsibility for patient management in order for them to experience the satisfaction and excitement of coping with complex geriatric problems.

Holtzman, et al. [2,3] have shown that different types of geriatric programs can have differing degrees of effect on students. Experiences based entirely within the nursing home had little effect on student attitudes, whereas a deliberate empathy-raising experience, including exposure to the well elderly with little emphasis on the institutionalized elderly, had a demonstrably positive effect.

Does the responsibility for the teaching of geriatrics need to rest within any of the traditional departments? There are several gerontology programs without a definite affiliation with one particular clinical department. It might be ideal if an independent office of gerontology within a medical school established liaison with the relevant personnel in the appropriate departments ensuring emphasis on geriatric medicine at all levels of the curriculum. However, if interested clinical faculty exist in a particular department, such as family practice, internal medicine, or psychiatry, then having one such department concentrate on geriatrics would ensure that students had credible role models, and would be able to observe physicians working in an enthusiastic and comprehensive way with the elderly.

One means of determining the content of the geriatric curriculum for students was addressed in a contract (Development of a Model Geriatrics Curriculum in Medical School Undergraduate Primary Care Education, Health Resources Administration Contract No. 232-79-0111) awarded to the American Geriatrics Society and subcontracted to Southern Illinois University School of Medicine. Under this contract, an attempt is being made to develop a model curriculum in geriatric primary care for medical students. The areas of primary-care geriatrics that are presently omitted from most medical school curricula have been defined. Instructional units are based on these defined areas of "core material." The instructional material is problem oriented and uses clinical cases. Thus, the student will be encouraged to bring about the best possible resolution of such problems with a maximum of independence and a minimum of iatrogenic illness. This curriculum, when completed, will enable students to have a systematic approach in mind when seeing elderly patients and will foster the right blend of optimism and realism in therapy and rehabilitation.

Increased emphasis on geriatrics as a primary-care endeavor at the residency level is also of considerable importance. House officers will inevitably interact with large numbers of elderly patients and will frequently function as primary-care physicians, even if their specialty is not one of those defined as such. The emphasis must be on psychological and social content as well as the physical aspects of geriatric medicine.

A number of persons have done work on the appropriate content of family practice residencies. Pattee [7], Moore and Kane [8], Kelly [9], and others have attempted to define what family practice residents should know. Departments of Family Practice not based on existing practices will initially tend to attract younger patients. Establishing a focus of interest in geriatrics within a department will help to increase the geriatric population served.

These remarks are not intended to be confined to family medicine residencies. If an internal medicine program is attempting to develop primary-care internists, then the same aspects of geriatric medicine should be covered. Furthermore, development of special fellowships in geriatric medicine must not allow a relaxation of our efforts to incorporate geriatrics into all primary-care residency programs.

Experience with senior citizen centers, day care units, hospices, skilled nursing-care facilities, retirement communities, and home health-care services should occur early in any residency training program for primary-care physicians. Furthermore, residents should be able to work with nurse practitioners, physician assistants, homemakers, home health aides, and service providers. Setting up such experiences for residents is not difficult as medical input is usually welcome by most services to the elderly.

Of special relevance to the teaching of primary-care geriatrics is continuing medical education (CME). Such an experience must ensure that:

1. New information in this dynamic and changing field is disseminated to all the appropriate physicians.

2. Appropriate attitudes and interests in all practicing physicians dealing with the elderly be encouraged.
3. Proper use of and collaboration with other health professionals and a host of psychosocial services be promoted.

The Report from the Institute of Medicine [10] on the incorporation of geriatrics into medical education noted that only a minute proportion of all CME courses were specifically concerned with geriatrics. Recently, the number has risen, but geriatrics is still poorly represented. Most CME programs make use of formal lectures. In the teaching of geriatrics, where individual attitudes and the approach to the patient are so important, it can be more beneficial to make use of small group discussions.

Studies by Stross and Harlan [11,12] clearly demonstrate some of the difficulties in communicating new medical information; yet, material relevant to geriatric care must be incorporated into CME programs of a general nature, especially those designed for internists and family physicians [13,14]. Indeed, it may be more beneficial to incorporate geriatrics into "general" types of CME courses than into "all geriatric" courses.

Older physicians tend to work in areas with proportionately larger populations of elderly persons [15]; they often rely on drug detail persons to obtain new information [12]. Clearly, this system will tend to overemphasize drug treatment when alternatives might be available. Self-study, credit-earning materials for use by practicing physicians are now offered by a number of organizations and can be especially useful for isolated primary-care practitioners.

The problem of how to make better use of journals for the training of practicing primary-care physicians needs to be addressed. In one survey, an important medical fact relevant to physicians treating diabetics failed to be noted appropriately because it was published in an ophthalmologic journal [11]. Thus, it is essential to incorporate information about advances in geriatric medicine into appropriate journals actually read by physicians.

Textbooks are widely used, especially by younger physicians [12]. Several textbooks of geriatric medicine have recently been published [16,17,18], but there is still a need for a briefer review, revised annually, emphasizing recent advances in the field. A potential model has been developed in the United Kingdom as well as brief texts that can be useful for practicing physicians [19,20,21].

Finally, one specific teaching tool needs to be mentioned. To help those involved in the primary care of the elderly understand the impact of visual and auditory losses and the impact of changes in environment, visual and auditory distortion equipment can be used. These materials will increase individual empathy and sensitivity and will result in more sympathetic handling of, and effective communication with, older patients.

An important method for reaching physicians at all levels, which is especially useful in the training and coordination of care with other health professionals, is the interdisciplinary conference. Such conferences, focusing on one patient or one type of problem, can bring in all of those involved in the patient's care. Teamwork is promoted and health professionals come to understand one another's roles. It is striking to notice how misinformed some practicing physicians are about the training and background of other health-care professionals.

Physicians in geriatric medicine, especially those offering primary care, must be involved in the training of other health professionals. Physician assistants, nurse practitioners, nurses, social workers, volunteers, and many others who come into contact with the elderly all require instruction. Furthermore, primary-care physicians should learn from nurses and others, for it is they and not the doctors who spend the most time with the patient and, thus, have the most intimate knowledge of patient needs and concerns.

Medical directors of long-term-care facilities play a potentially significant role in education, patient care, rehabilitation, and, perhaps, the discouragement of unnecessary institutionalization of the elderly. Educational opportunities specifically directed to the needs of this group need to be arranged.

The teaching of primary-care geriatrics must take place in a variety of settings, at all levels of medical education, and for all types of health care professionals. The health care problems of the elderly must be seen in positive yet realistic terms. The interaction of psychological, social, and physical problems in the production of functional disability must be understood. The use of a variety of modes of therapy, and of other health-care professionals, as well as all possible community and home-care resources to promote the independent, healthy functioning of old people must be encouraged. New information relevant to geriatric medicine must be communicated in the most effective and attractive way possible so that busy practicing primary-care physicians have access to the information in a form that will encourage its use in their practices. Only by working on the knowledge and attitudes of physicians and other health-care professionals at all levels of their training can improvements in geriatric primary care be obtained and sustained.

References

1. Coggan, P., Hodgetts, P., Holtzman, J., Ryan, N., and Ham, R. A required program in geriatrics for medical students. *J. Fam. Pract.* 7(4):735, 1978.

2. Holtzman, J., Beck, J., Hodgetts, P., Coggan, P., and Ryan, N. Geriatrics program for medical students and family practice residents. I. Establishing attitudes toward the aged. *J. Am. Geriatrics Soc.* 11:521, 1977.

3. Holtzman, J., Beck, J., and Coggan, P. Geriatrics program for medical students. II. The impact of two educational experiences on student attitudes. *J. Am. Geriatrics Soc.* 8:355, 1978.

4. Gale, J., and Livesley, B. Attitudes towards geriatrics: A report of the King's Survey. *Age and Aging* 7:49, 1974.

5. Miller, D., Lowenstein, R., and Winston, R. Physicians' attitudes towards the ill aged and nursing homes. *J. Am. Geriatrics. Soc.* 24:497, 1976.

6. Spence, D., Feigenbaum, E., Fitzgerald, F., and Roth, J. Medical students' attitudes toward the geriatric patient. *J. Am. Geriatrics Soc.* 16:976, 1968.

7. Pattee, J. Training objectives of a well developed geriatric program. *J. Am. Geriatrics Soc.* 4:167, 1978.

8. Moore, J. and Kane, W. Geriatrics training in family medicine: The natural history of a developing program. *J. Fam. Pract.* 1:79, 1979.

9. Kelly, J.T., et al. An operational model for teaching geriatric medicine in a family practice residency program. *J. Fam. Pract.* 4:1103, 1977.

10. Aging and medical education. Report of a study. Institute of Medicine. Natural Academy of Science, Washington, D.C., Sept. 1978.

11. Stross, J.K. and Harlan, W.R. The dissemination of new medical information. JAMA 241(24):2622, 1979.

12. Stross, J.K. and Harlan, W.R. The impact of mandatory continuing education. JAMA 239(25):2663, 1978.

13. Mendenhall, R.C., Girard, R.A., Lloyd, J.S., et al. Internal medicine practice study report (USE/DRMED-1055), Division of Research in Medical Education, USC School of Medicine, Los Angeles, California, 1978.

14. Mendenhall, R.C., Girard, R.A., Lloyd, J.S., et al. Family practice study report (USE/DRMED-1085), Division of Research in Medical Education, USC School of Medicine, Los Angeles, California, 1978.

15. Silvertson, S.E., et al. The relation between physician and patient age in family practice. *J. Fam. Pract.* 3:305, 1978.

16. Reichel, W. (Ed.). *Clinical Aspects of Aging.* Baltimore, Md.: Williams and Wilkins, 1978.

17. Reichel, W. (Ed.) *The Geriatric Patient.* New York: Hospital Practice, 1978.

18. Rossman, I. *Clinical Geriatrics* (2nd ed.). Philadelphia, Penn.: Lippincott, 1979.

19. *Recent Advances in Geriatrics I and II.* New York: Churchill Livingston, 1980.

20. Coni, N., Davison, W., and Webster, S. *Lecture Notes on Geriatrics.* Oxford, England: Blackwell, 1977.

21. Brocklehurst, J.C. and Hanley, T. *Geriatric Medicine for Students.* New York; Churchill Livingston, 1976.

18 Establishing An Academic Unit in Geriatric Medicine —An Internist's Point of View

Evan Calkins, M.D.

The growing challenge, in this country and in all developed countries, to provide appropriate care for older citizens has been well documented. So, too, has the high cost of the pattern of care that we presently provide for this segment of our population. The fact that the 10% of our citizens, aged 65 and over, account for the expenditure of nearly 33% of present health-care dollars may or may not be inappropriate in itself [1]. What is of greater concern is that the segment of this population that is in the greatest need of care, those aged 75 and older, will substantially increase over the next ten years [2]. To an increasing extent, society in general and, especially, the progressively well-educated "young old" (those aged 55 through 75) are questioning whether this money is being well spent. Is the system through which we provide medical and social support to older people designed to meet their needs in a cost-efficient manner? The answer would appear to be no.

The fact that these problems will be of even greater concern to future providers of care leads to an equally urgent question. Are the educational patterns and priorities of our present medical school faculty appropriately designed to equip our students to respond to these needs? Here, again, the answer is quite clearly no.

How does one go about setting up an academic unit in geriatric medicine? There are, I believe, four functional requirements of a teaching unit in this field. The first three of these are the legs of the "three legged stool" so often referred to by academic internists: patient care, teaching, and research.

Patient Care

Central to the effectiveness of an academic unit in geriatric medicine is that it must be based on an effective clinical unit or activity. This should be so designed that it will constitute a significant and identifiable presence within one of the major teaching units of the medical school, preferably the university hospital. These two statements contain a number of individual components, each of which merit consideration and each of which is, in my view, important.

First, let us consider the connotations of the term "clinical unit." There has been sharp disagreement within departments of medicine concerning whether the teaching unit should "have its own beds." Alternatively, should the inpatient wards be established as *general* medical services, to which the members of various subspecialty groups serve as consultants? In the case of geriatric medicine, it is my view that the unit should include direct responsibility for a segment of inpatient medicine—"have its own beds." These can be acute-care beds, possibly established as a diagnostic or assessment unit, or they may be intermediate-care beds, or both. Assignment of responsibility for patients awaiting placement in a nursing home does not represent an appropriate response to this need.

There are at least two reasons why, in my view, a geriatric medicine unit should include responsibility for geographically defined geriatric beds. The first relates to the need for academic physicians to obtain personal experience in clinical geriatric medicine. One of the problems of this field is that, within this country, there are far too few knowledgeable and experienced teachers. In a long-established specialty, such as cardiology or endocrinology, a trainee or fellow has the opportunity to learn from his or her preceptors, as well as from the patients. In geriatric medicine, however, the faculty must "learn as they go." The only way to do this is by assuming direct responsibility for the care of the patients.

It is evident that continuity of care is one of the essential elements of geriatric medicine. One can never derive a true understanding of this field if responsibility for the care of patients during a particular phase of illness, such as an acute hospitalization or home care, is delegated to others. The academic geriatric physician must be in charge of his or her patients through the entire spectrum of care. To be maximally effective, such a unit should have geographic and administrative integrity, since both are essential for maximal development of the multidisciplinary team. The multiplicity of needs in the elderly cannot be taken care of if each professional is directly responsible to the appropriate service chief (chief of medicine, director of nursing or social work, and so on). Instead, direct responsibility should be vested in a unit chief, who will coordinate the activities of professionals of all disciplines that are assigned to the service.

The above comments focus on the inpatient service because this is the area in which the greatest controversy is apt to occur. It is evident, however, that comprehensive continuing care of older people involves the whole continuum, including ambulatory or office practice, home care, day care, and long-term institutional care, in addition to acute care and evaluation. If possible, the team of physicians, social workers, and nurse practitioners should follow individual patients throughout this continuum.

In stressing the importance of a geriatric acute-care or assessment unit, I do not mean to suggest that a geriatrics service should attempt to provide care for all older patients within the institution, whether on an inpatient or outpatient basis. The number of patients should be limited to those necessary for teaching, clinical experience, and research, and for appropriate participation in the ongoing clinical responsibilities of the hospital. In addition, the geriatrics unit should maintain an active consultation service.

With regard to the institutional location of the geriatric unit, it seems probable that the concepts described above can be established more easily in a peripheral or affiliated institution, rather than at the major teaching hospital. The disadvantage of such an arrangement, however, is that it conveys to students and house staff the impression that geriatric medicine is not a high-priority area. Since geriatrics needs to attract the interest and attention of the best of our students, it cannot be perceived as being a second-rate specialty. At the University of Rochester, where an ideal arrangement for this kind of a program exists at the Monroe Community Hospital (not the major teaching hospital), special attention has been given to emphasizing the priority of this program by including the medical director of the hospital on the executive committee of the medical school and by initiating regularly scheduled rotations of house staff among all relevant medical specialties [3].

Teaching

Many would urge, with some logic, that teaching should be cited as the first objective of an academic program. Nevertheless, it is my belief that an effective teaching program cannot be assembled from lectures and seminars organized by people who are not themselves involved in geriatric medicine but must be based on personal experience in a functioning geriatrics unit.

The teaching program should be multifaceted, including preceptorial teaching to students as part of their initial medical school experience; well-organized curricular offerings in the physiological, biochemical, and behavioral aspects of aging; clinical programs for senior medical students and house staff; participation with the faculty of the schools of nursing, social work, allied health, and pharmacy in curricular offerings to students in these disciplines; and a variety of programs in continuing education. This is a big order for a division or program that will probably be small, at least initially. Priorities must be established.

The most important initial target of the teaching program should be the medical house staff. In settings in which it is appropriate, this should also include the house staff in family medicine. After seventeen years of experience as chief of medicine of a large student and house staff teaching program, I have been impressed with the fact that the most important and effective opinion makers and teachers of medical students are not the faculty but their slightly older contemporaries, the house staff. A negative attitude is almost inevitably encountered among medical house staff toward the older patients who flood the teaching services in increasing numbers. These feelings of antagonism and resentment among the house staff are a result of a perception by them that they are being "used by the system." They resent it and this resentment is contagious among the students, resulting in unhumanistic feelings by many students during their early medical school years. In developing a teaching program directed toward the house staff, we have followed the concept that one reason for their resentment stems from the fact that the house staff are not taught about the unique problems presented by older patients, and the modalities available to meet these problems. We postulate that if the house staff could be shown that logical therapeutic approaches are available and that management of these patients can convey a personal sense of achievement and gratification for the physician involved, at least some of this resentment can be abated and, hopefully, replaced by enthusiasm.

In the development of the teaching program at our insitution we have concentrated, initially, in clinical pharmacology. Through a cooperative arrangement with the chairman of the department of pharmacology and a junior faculty member, we have initiated bimonthly clinical pharmacology rounds on the intermediate-care service at the VA Medical Center. Attended by the fellows in geriatric medicine, myself, the nurse practitioner, medical students on elective rotation and, frequently, the head nurse, these sessions have proved to be informative and stimulating. We have come to realize the extent to which the problems arising on the service stem from inappropriate use of drugs. In the next phase of our development, we are "opening up" a small number of acute-care geriatric beds as a component of one of the general medical teaching services. We are confident that the input from the clinical pharmacology group will prove as enlightening to the medical house staff as it has to us and will constitute one step in the development of a positive image for geriatric medicine among the house staff.

Other aspects of medicine, equally important to patients in the geriatric age group and almost completely overlooked by the traditional teaching service as presently constituted, are the areas of liaison psychiatry, rehabilitation medicine, and home care. (A liaison psychiatrist has just joined our team, and is relating both to the acute and intermediate care services.)

Research

Funds for research in the field of geriatric medicine are beginning to be available through the National Institute on Aging and other sources. Surely it would be foolish to define geriatric medicine as the one branch of medical science that does not require good research. Participation in this effort is a necessary component of a good academic geriatric program.

Community Involvement

To the classic legs of the three-legged stool described above, one must add, in the case of geriatric medicine, a fourth leg—community involvement. Geriatrics is the one branch of medicine that is most ill-suited to the setting of the tertiary care hospital, with its many rather-circumscribed subspecialty units and clinics and its tradition of fragmented care. It is increasingly clear that an important goal of geriatric medicine is to keep older people at home. This is recognized in New York State, for example, through the development of the "nursing home without walls." It is reinforced by my own experience, with my parents, and with a growing list of older patients. This does not mean that there is no place for long-term institutional care; however, there is a great need for the creation of settings in which multidisciplinary comprehensive care can be provided and taught outside of the framework of the traditional hospital or long-term-care facility.

This creates special problems for the physician interested in the teaching of geriatric medicine. Because of the recent advances in biomedical science and increasing reliance on complex diagnostic and therapeutic modalities, the hospital has emerged as the setting in which medical education can most easily take place. Everything is at hand—records, laboratory support, consultants, and a fiscal structure that has fostered the use of hospitals as the proper setting for diagnosis and treatment. Few of these advantages are at hand for a teaching program in the home or community. The system of care is fragmented and disorganized, and the fiscal arrangements complex and often inadequate. This, in turn creates a situation in which the physician interested in developing good settings for geriatric education must be an opportunist and an activist. Direct and active involvement in community affairs becomes inescapable.

This review of the essential elements of an academic program in geriatric medicine leads to the consideration of the truly formidable problems that must be faced to develop an effective academic program in geriatric medicine. How can one possibly accomplish this broad range of objectives, in what must be regarded as one of the low earning specialties, in which recruitment of competent staff continues to present a problem? Unfortunately, I cannot yet offer a confident answer, although three principles are beginning to emerge from my experience so far.

The first is that one cannot possibly attempt to establish a creditable academic program without a team. This should include a minimum of four full-time faculty, preferably twice that number. At least one of these should have an active commitment in research; one should emphasize community relationships; one clinical teaching; and one, preferably the director, overall administration. In addition, the unit should include at least one multidisciplinary clinical team, including representatives of the full range of health-related specialties concerned with long-term care.

Second, one cannot create and maintain a team of this sort without appropriate institutional support. With the current framework of health-care financing, this can probably be achieved only as a result of assuming responsibility for an inpatient service in a VA hospital or other institution that maintains responsibility for ongoing care. The setting should be selected carefully so that the academic needs and goals, including those of research, will not be suffocated by service demands.

Finally, in selecting personal goals, the director of a geriatrics unit must value time above all else. The day is not long enough to permit the director to participate equally in all of the cited activities. Care must be taken to identify which activity represents the most appropriate time investment at a given period in the development of the program. In the last analysis, if the director is forced to identify one aspect of academic life that cannot be sacrificed, I believe that continued effectiveness as a good physician is the one characteristic that is the most essential for a satisfactory outcome.

References

1. Corman, J.C. Health services for the elderly. In *Sourcebook on Aging* (1st Ed.). Chicago, Ill.: Marquis Academic Media, Marquis Who's Who, Inc., 1977.

2. Neugarten, B.L. and Havighurst, R.J. Aging and the Future. In *Sourcebook on Aging* (1st Ed.). Marquis Academic Media, Marquis Who's Who, Inc., 1977.

3. Williams, T.F., Izzo, A.J., and Steel, R.K. Innovations in teaching about chronic illness and aging in a chronic disease hospital. In D.W. Clark and T.F. Williams (Eds.) *Teaching of Chronic Illness and Aging.* Bethesda, Md.: The Fogarty International Center, NIH, 1976.

19

The British Geriatric System: What Can We Learn from their Efforts?

David K. Carboni, Ph.D.

The British National Health Service (NHS) differs from the American health-care delivery system in significant ways. Therefore, British experiences in geriatric care are not immediately transferable to the American scene. Nevertheless, the NHS has attempted to respond in an organized fashion to the needs of the chronically ill aged over the past thirty years and much can be learned from their experiences.

Before discussing current issues in British geriatric care, I think it would be useful to discuss the historical development of British geriatrics since the inception of the NHS. This review provides a context for contemporary issues in geriatric care and reminds us that any system of comprehensive geriatric care must be consistent with existing medical care patterns in a given country.

Britain nationalized virtually all hospitals with the establishment of the NHS in 1947. With very few exceptions, physicians who became specialist consultants received salaries and practiced exclusively in district general hospitals. Doctors who entered general practice continued to practice outside the major hospitals, meeting the primary-care needs of patients in the community. The NHS contracted with these individuals on a per-capita basis. That is, the general practitioners (GPs) received a fixed stipend for each person under care. Except for smaller community hospitals in outlying regions, the GP did not have admitting privileges to hospitals. Therefore, the GP relinquished to the consultant the care of a patient when the individual was admitted to the hospital, and reassumed these responsibilities upon discharge.

From the earliest days of the NHS, caring for the chronically ill aged presented the Ministry of Health, the central policy-making body of the NHS, with severe problems. Inadequately staffed geriatric hospitals, often located in former poor houses and poor law infirmaries, came under the direct responsibility of the Ministry of Health. Their task was to encourage the development of appropriate administrative arrangements in order to meet the needs of the chronically ill aged residing in geriatric wards. The solution had to be acceptable to the medical profession because, without their support, any comprehensive policy directed to improving geriatric care would fail.

Early efforts in British geriatrics provided principles of care that served to shape the character of geriatric services in the United Kingdom. One of the notable individuals of this pioneering period during the mid-1930s was Dr. Marjory Warren who assumed the task of managing the chronically ill of a large poor law infirmary that had been absorbed by the West Middlesex Hospital. She began by carefully examining each patient under her charge and developing care plans appropriate for the conditions she uncovered [1]. To her colleagues' surprise, she discovered many remediable conditions in patients previously thought to be irremediable. Dr. Warren's discharge rate reached 25%, a level much in excess of that achieved by other facilities for the chronic sick at that time [2]. Dr. Warren instilled a new feeling of therapeutic optimism.

At about the same time, Dr. Lionel Cosin, the Medical Superintendent at Orsett in Essex, proposed that elderly patients with fractured hips be approached surgically, and he insisted on early and thorough mobilization following surgery. Many of his patients recovered rapidly and resumed walking, which allowed them to return to their homes [2]. This principle of early mobilization was later applied to patients with a variety of illnesses. In general, patients were encouraged to be out of bed at the earliest possible time.

Dr. Eric Brooke encouraged the development of geriatric medicine by supporting the need for the home visit. With a limited number of hospital beds under his charge, increasing numbers of older persons filled his waiting list for admission. Under considerable pressure from general practitioners, other community-health professionals and relatives of the elderly patients, Brooke attempted to rectify the situation by visiting those who were awaiting admission [2]. As geriatricians were later to recognize, he noted that many older persons had a complicated web of medical and social problems. In some cases, he was able to mobilize community support services to meet their needs so that hospitalization became unnecessary. Home visiting, then, reduced waiting lists for admission and increased the efficiency of serving the ill elderly of the district.

Geriatrics as a separate specialty was introduced by the Ministry of Health as a sort of experiment, and the number of geriatric departments established in the ten years following World War II remained small [3]. In about 1960, the Ministry of Health became convinced of the need for geriatrics as a separate specialty within the NHS. Since that time, the number of consultant posts has more than tripled and at present there exists over 350 posts. The first formal posts for training in geriatrics by senior registrars were also created at that time. The decision to encourage the growth of geriatrics, then, was an administrative decision by the Ministry of Health. It did not reflect the attitudes of the health-care profession as a whole and there may still be some resentment by general medicine toward the growth of geriatrics.

British geriatricians argue that there are unique clinical and socioclinical problems for geriatric patients. Often noted are the nonclassical presentation of symptoms ("silent" heart attacks) and changing norms for a host of physiologic parameters (alterations in the blood pressure with aging). Furthermore, British geriatricians stress the profound interaction of psychiatric and physical symptoms that accompany illness in the aged as compared with younger persons. They also point up the influence of social and economic problems on the physical presentation of illness. Other issues that tend to set geriatric medicine apart are the frequent multiplicity of chronic diseases and disabilities in elderly persons and the need for the use of multiple pharmacologic agents in the same in-individual raising the risks associated with such "poly-pharmacy" [4].

British geriatricians argue that the often unique clinical and socioclinical problems presented by geriatric patients necessitate a special approach to management of the elderly patient. Disability must be recognized as being of great concern in geriatric illness. Indeed, the dysfunction can require evaluation and treatment distinct from the underlying disease processes. Thus, most geriatricians emphasize that they continue to be involved with the rehabilitation of their patients, even after the acute aspects of illness have stabilized. This often requires close contact with the community-health team.

When considering the NHS, it is easy to assume that a centrally imposed monolithic health-care system can accommodate itself only poorly to varying local conditions and needs. This is not the case. There remains an "ideal" system of geriatric care in Great Britain, but is is interpreted differently and applied unevenly throughout the country. It includes:

1. *Geriatric assessment beds* in the District General Hospital, which are controlled by a consultant geriatrician and where complex problems of geriatric patients are diagnosed and evaluated.

2. *Rehabilitation beds* where short-term rehabilitation occurs and continuing care plans for geriatric patients are developed. Usually the rehabilitation stay is about two to three weeks.

3. *Long-stay beds* which, as the name implies, are for those geriatric patients who are unable to return to their homes.

All of these beds are under the direction of the geriatric department of the district general hospital, and the consultant geriatrician can move patients to different levels of care as required, with the GP sharing clinical responsibilities for geriatric patients in long-stay wards in many parts of the country.

The team care provided outside the hospital, directed by the GP, consists of the district nurse, social worker, health visitor, and, if needed, home help. Since group practices of GPs are common now in many parts of Britain, the health-care team may be large. The GP retains responsibility for this care system, seeking consultation from the consultant geriatrician only on very complicated cases. Thus, as noted by Ashworth, "It is the GP's responsibility to see that all forces are mobilized to keep the geriatric patient healthy and happy at home" [5]. The theme of geriatric medicine for the primary-care provider is seen in the observation of Forsyth and Logan, who concluded that "it is the general practitioner who is required to accept continuing responsibility for the care of the elderly, not only in prevention and delaying the onset and progress of disease, but also in postponing disability and delaying handicap" [6].

Nonetheless, there are serious problems in the system of geriatric care as developed under the NHS. Perhaps the most notable difficulty is centered around the divisions of care to the elderly between the GP and the consultant. It may not be possible for the GP to offer the type of service required for the geriatric patient without the support of the geriatric department, particularly in rehabilitation. There may be a conflict over who should assume continuing care responsibility for the geriatric patient. Because there are no explicit guidelines for professional role relationships between the geriatrician and the GP, dividing professional responsibilities tends to be negotiated at the local level. Other ambiguous areas of responsibility continue to be:

1. The designation of a responsible physician in certain circumstances. Thus, which physician (the GP or the geriatrician) is to assume continuing responsibility for the long-term-care patient, particularly the very-handicapped patient with poor prospects of returning to the community?

2. The prescribing of medication in certain circumstances. When a geriatric patient is discharged from the hospital where he has been under the care of the geriatrician a group of drugs may be ordered. Unaware of the hospital prescription, the GP may prescribe additional drugs upon reassuming care of the patient.

3. The follow-up care of geriatric patients discharged from one hospital carried out in another setting. Thus, in some cases, the GP leaves follow-up care of the discharged geriatric patient to the hospital geriatric department. These patients will then be seen periodically by the geriatric department, but rarely seen by the GP [3], who may have previously functioned as the primary-care provider.

A second difficulty with the way geriatrics is managed by the NHS is one of inadequate resources. Other problems in British geriatric care are linked directly or indirectly to insufficient funds, particularly when compared with resources allocated to general medicine departments. This inequality has a number of negative consequences.

Inadequate monies and facilities for the geriatric department leads to low status for geriatrics within the hospital, which in turn, makes it difficult to attract high quality recruits to this area of medical care. In fact, British geriatric medicine has faced recruitment problems throughout its brief history, although some of these problems are caused by the rapid expansion of the specialty. Thus, some believe there is a two-tier system of care in Britain—one for those not yet old, and one for geriatric patients [7]. Clearly such inequity in the distribution of money and facilities can lead to morale problems among staff. Health professionals become discouraged when they are not provided with the care resources needed to clinically manage the aged ill and disabled patients under their charge.

The positive aspects of British geriatrics center around the principles they have applied to the care designed to meet the needs of the multi-problem elderly patient. Although some of these principles are not applicable to the American scene, others are. Geriatric medicine, as it develops in the United States, must consider:

1. How to build incentives into the system so as to encourage the maintenance of the older person in the home.

2. How to adapt the British system of geriatric-care facilities that allows relatively free movement of patients along the continuum of care as changing needs warrant.

3. How to most effectively use the British health-care team approach, which is for them a *sine qua non* of effectively managing multi-problem geriatric patients.

4. How care modalities, such as the day hospital, adult day care center, and holiday respite hospitalization for support system relief, all supportive of a comprehensive geriatric health-care system, might be adopted here.

5. How to develop a preventive-care program. The British geriatric care stresses the importance of seeking out unreported illness among the elderly so as not to overwhelm the care system with crisis care.

It is equally important to learn from Britain's mistakes. It would indeed be unfortunate to establish a two-tier system of geriatric care in the United States, as some critics suggest the British system has done. By separating geriatric departments from mainstream medicine, British geriatric patients have not had access to the resources that medical wards provide. Furthermore, British geriatric care has evolved within a system of care that has traditionally blocked the general practitioner from following patients into the hospital. As discussed earlier, this had led to problems associated with the ambiguities inherent in this sort of divided care.

For any system of geriatric care to be effective, it must be consistent with the strengths inherent in that country's medical-care system. To artificially transplant British geriatric-care systems to the United States would be fruitless. We must take what is best from their system, modify it to suit our needs, and apply it according to local requirements and circumstances. To do otherwise would not be in the interests of American geriatric patients who deserve the best care possible.

References

1. Warren, M. Care of chronic aged sick. *Lancet* 1:841, 1946.

2. Howell, T. Comment: Origins of the British geriatrics society. *Age and Aging* 3(2):68, 1974.

3. Carboni, D.K. Occupational specialization movements: The case of geri-

atric medicine in Great Britain and the USA. Unpublished doctoral dissertation, Univ. of Conn., p. 162, 1979.

4. Special Committee on Geriatric Services. *Planning and Organization of Geriatric Services.* Technical Report Series No. 548. Geneva: World Health Organization, 1974.

5. Ashworth, H.W. *Medical World* 91:314, 1959.

6. Forsyth, G. and Logan, R.E.L. *J. Chronic Dis.* 17:789, 1964.

7. Leonard, J.C. Should geriatrics survive? *Brit. Med. J.* 1 (6021): 1335, 1976.

20 Ambulatory Geriatric Care —A National Perspective

Jon C. Calvert, M.D., Ph.D.
Hugo K. Koch M.H.A.

Health care for the elderly and the education and training of health professionals in the care of the elderly is receiving increased emphasis in this country, an emphasis that is long overdue. Surveys of geriatric education published in the early 60s and 70s are being augmented in the medical education literature with other articles that discuss the state of geriatric education as well as issues of attitude and curriculum design and content for medical students, residents, fellows, and practicing physicians. The question of whether or not there should be a specialty of geriatrics and/or gerontology is being considered [1].

As teachers of geriatric medicine, one of our responsibilities is to determine content and instructional methodology. Understanding the needs and demographics of the population served is central to this process. Some have observed that our hospital-based medical school and residency training programs produce physicians who have a better understanding of acute, hospital-based geriatric care than of ambulatory and nursing home care of the elderly [1]. Over the past seven years we have noted that our residents tend to apply hospital-based expectations, attitudes, and knowledge to their continuing care of a panel of nursing home and ambulatory elderly. This generally results in feelings of frustration as well as feelings of inadequacy and insecurity when these efforts meet with resistance or failure. These expectations, developed during medical school and internship, must be reshaped to meet the needs of the ambulatory and nursing home elderly. Fortunately, there are data now available to help us delineate the specific health-care needs of these different groups of patients. This will direct medical educators to develop balanced instructional programs for medical students, residents, fellows, and practicing physicians, programs which properly prepare physicians to care for the elderly in the hospital, the long-term-care facility, the office, and the patient's home.

In the early 1970s, the National Center for Health Statistics began gathering and publishing data on ambulatory health care [2-18]. Review of these and other published data provides a revealing picture of the dimensions of the ambulatory health care needs of the 65 and older population, which in turn will allow for guidelines for the development of geriatric training in the primary care specialties.

Why the increased interest in geriatric health care? It is well known and accepted that in the future the elderly will comprise an increasingly larger percentage of our total population [1]. With this growth, increasing demands will be placed on private health-care resources and the family, as well as on community, state and federal resources. Demands for support services will continue to be out of proportion to the relative size of the elderly population.

Geriatric education and training in American schools of medicine has not met the needs of the public. In 1976, only 32 of 114 schools of medicine offered courses in geriatrics (compared to 10 of 16 Canadian schools) [1]. In addition, existing geriatric training has been limited to and focused on acute hospital care to the exclusion of a balanced curriculum to include the elderly patient in other settings. Functional assessment, long-term management of multiple problems, physical therapy, and the identification and management of medical and social resources, skills frequently used in outpatient care of the elderly, may not be stressed or taught at all.

Primary-care physicians are aware that most care of the elderly does not take place in the setting of the acute hospital or even the nursing home. Most elderly are ambulatory and are provided care in the physician's office. Data gathered by the National Center for Health Statistics supports this observation [2-18]. In 1977, approximately 5% of all persons 65 and older resided in long-term-care facilities [1]. Approximately the same percentage were occupying a bed in an an acute hospital setting. This means that, on any given day in 1977, 90% of the nation's elderly population were potential candidates for noninstitutionalized or ambulatory care.

Of these 21.5 million ambulatory elderly, 54% live with a spouse [1]. This represents over 5 million husband and wife family units. Approximately 4 million elderly (19%) live with someone other than a spouse. There are over 6 million persons (29%) who live alone. This group especially requires ongoing functional assessment [1].

When in need of ambulatory care, the elderly sought it chiefly in the physician's office where 77% of all outpatient physician contacts occurred. Telephone conversations accounted for another 9% and 9% occurred in outpatient clinics and emergency rooms. Home visits by physicians accounted for only 1.5%. (Unpublished data from the Health Interview Survey, National Center for Health Statistics, 1977).

Clearly, then, most geriatric care is ambulatory and most of this ambulatory care takes place in the physician's office. One national survey of such office-based care produced an estimated 92 million visits made by elderly patients in 1977, an average of just over four visits per elderly person per year, when the national average was 2.7 visits per person per year [5].

It would surprise most medical students to know that 29% of the ambulatory elderly consider themselves to be in excellent health and another 40% consider themselves in good health. Only 9% consider themselves in poor health [1]. Thus, medical students, residents, and practicing health professionals who do not encounter the ambulatory elderly on a continuing basis fail to appreciate that most older persons do not think of themselves as ill.

Eighty-five percent of elderly persons can identify a regular source of care, which is utilized in a consistent and continuing manner [3]. Of those who could not identify a source of care, over 50% stated that they had no need for a physician; 7% could not find a physician; and 9% had a physician who was currently not available. The task of getting an appointment or finding an available doctor was no more difficult for the elderly than any other age group. However, this age group found physical access to medical care twice as difficult as other age groups. For the elderly, lack of suitable transportation is a more significant barrier to medical care than identification or availability of a physician [3].

The office practice pattern of care for the elderly differs from that of younger patient populations. For every new elderly patient seen in a physician's office, there were two new younger patients seen. Seventy-six percent of elderly encounters were return visits for previously identified problems. Fewer than 16% of these visits were for a new problem [9]. Two out of every three visits were for a chronic or continuing problem. Although relatively fewer in number, when compared with younger age groups, acute problems in the elderly population tended to restrict activity for longer periods of time [9]. When physicians were asked to classify the seriousness of the patient's problem, they stated that two of three office visits by an elderly patient were for a serious or very serious problem, whereas less than 50% of the visits in the younger population were considered serious [9].

On a per visit basis, the physician spends more time with the elderly patient than with the younger population. For the 65 and older group, 27% of the visits lasted six to ten minutes (compared to 32% for the younger population); 31% lasted eleven to fifteen minutes (compared to 26% for the younger population). For the geriatric patient, approximately 25% of the visits lasted 16 to 30 minutes (compared to 18% for the younger population). There is increasing time spent with the elderly even though nine of ten patients in this group had been seen previously. For the elderly, physician-to-patient contact occurred in ninety-nine of every one hundred visits [9]. These are factors that increase the providers cost of rendering medical care.

Determination of activities that occur during an office visit speak not only to content of office visits but also to the kind of care provided. Data reveal that during 50% of the visits one or more of the following occurred: a prescription was written; a limited physical examination was carried out; a blood pressure check was completed; and/or a lab test or procedure was obtained.

Most patients seen have multiple problems. These problems differ from the younger age groups. Over 50% of the problems are related to one of four body systems: the circulatory system, the nervous system or sensory organs, the musculoskeletal system (including disorders of connective tissue), and the respiratory system [9]. For the elderly age group, the five most frequent ambulatory care diagnoses encountered were: essential benign hypertension; chronic ischemic heart disease; diabetes mellitus; medical and surgical after care; and osteoarthritis.

A study by Monroe underlines an equally important aspect of care in the 65 and older population—assessment of function [19]. This is of special importance in the area of continuing health-problem management of the elderly. Most primary-care physicians who have followed a patient and their family through the years are aware of details such as: where and with whom the patient lives; the patient's general economic situation; the patient's mental status and whether or not physical disability is present; and the patient's general ability to perform self care. This type of information is a bonus of continuous comprehensive care and is generally not accessible to episodic care givers. We believe that residents in training must have an opportunity to learn how to obtain and utilize functional assessment information.

In summary then, the typical geriatric patient is ambulatory; considers himself/herself to be in good or excellent health; has identified a source of care in the private sector (a source to which he continues to return); tends to have multiple and chronic problems; requires more time for recovery if afflicted with an acute illness; visits the physician's office more frequently; and spends a longer time with his physician, although the majority of visits are for the management of ongoing problems.

Finally, it must be noted that older patients see many types of doctors in the ambulatory setting. National Center for Health Statistics data gathered between 1974 and 1977 can be analyzed to determine both the percent of all visits made by the elderly population and the percent of each specialty visits made by those 65 years of age and over (see table 20-1). These data support the observation that there are disciplines other than internal medicine and family practice that made a significant contribution to the outpatient care of the elderly. Each of these other specialties should have training in geriatrics appropriate to their needs.

Awareness of these data for the ambulatory elderly as well as similar information for the acutely hospitalized elderly and the nursing home elderly is critical to the balanced educational and training curriculum for medical students and residents. The following should be considered when designing such curricula especially as they are developed for ambulatory care:

1. Emphasis should be given to the physiology of aging, functional assessment and interviewing skills, the management of a patient with multiple problems, how to utilize medical, family and community resources, and the prevention of illness.

2. The need to present the student with a balanced view of the elderly patient requires exposure to a variety of settings in which care can be provided.

3. The use of an interdisciplinary team should be available to students as most of the care of the elderly is provided by nonphysician members of health-care teams. The team should include members of the patient's family as well as the patient.

4. Specific faculty members who make excellent role models in the care of

Table 20-1
Office Visits for Aged 65 and Over by Specialty Area

Specialty	% All Visits[a]	% Specialty Visits	Survey Years[b]
Cardiovascular Specialist	3%	40%	1975–76
Chiropractic	–	4	1974
Dermatology	2	13	1975–76
General and Family Physician	46	18	1975
General Surgeon	8	18	1975
Internal Medicine	19	29	1975
Obstetrics and Gynecology	1	2	1975
Ophthalmologist	7	29	1975–76
Orthopedic surgeon	2	10	1975–76
Osteopath	–	19	1975
Otolaryngologist	2	14	1975–76
Physical Therapists	–	2	1974
Podiatrists	–	7	1974
Urology	3	28	1975–76

[a]Does not add up to exactly 100% as different years were analyzed.

[b]From National Center for Health Statistics.

the elderly patient should be identified. The individuals should be knowledgeable in the care of the geriatric patient, and they should demonstrate interest and enthusiasm for this care. They should not overtreat (the concept of minimal interference), but should assist the patient to maintain maximum independence. They must be individuals who are able to set realistic expectations, achieving gratification from accomplishments that may not be dramatic.

5. Ongoing analysis should be developed so that the product of instruction meets the patient's needs.

6. A plan to implement these goals must be one that is achievable. Moore and Kane have outlined their approach. It includes six steps: 1) involve students in the planning; 2) start with modest goals; 3) make programs relevant and practical; 4) build on local strengths; 5) include other health professional trainees; and 6) use ambulatory care, acute hospital care, and long-term care training sites [1].

The better we, as medical educators, understand the dimensions and needs of the population for whom our graduates are to provide health and medical services, the better we will be able to design educational and training programs for our students and residents.

References

1. Calvert, J.C. Care of the ambulatory elderly. In *Family Medicine Curriculum and Care of the Elderly*. J.G. O'Brien and A.C. Cunningham (Ed.). East Lansing, Michigan: Michigan State University, 1980.

2. Cypress, B.K. National ambulatory medical care survey of visits to general and family practitioners: United States, 1975. Advance Data, Vital and Health Statistics of the National Center of Health Statistics, U.S. DHEW, No. 15, December 14, 1977.

3. Drury, F. Access to ambulatory health care: United States, 1974. Advance Data, Vital and Health Statistics of the National Center for Health Statistics, U.S. DHEW, No. 17, February 23, 1978.

4. Cypress, B.K. Office visits to internists: National ambulatory medical care survey: United States. Advance Data, Vital and Health Statistics of the National Center for Health Statistics, U.S. DHEW, No. 16, February 7, 1978.

5. Ezzati, T. and McLenore, T. 1977 Summary: National ambulatory medical care survey. Advance Data, Vital and Health Statistics of the National Center for Health Statistics, U.S. DHEW, No. 48, April 13, 1979.

6. Ezzati, T. Office visits to dermatologists: National ambulatory medical care survey: United States, 1975-76. Advance Data, Vital and Health Statistics of the National Center for Health Statistics, U.S. DHEW No. 37, August 29, 1978.

7. Ezzati, T. Office visits to obstetricians and gynecologists: National ambulatory medical care survey: United States, 1975. Advance Data, Vital and Health Statistics of the National Center for Health Statistics, U.S. DHEW, No. 20, March 13, 1978.

8. Gagnon, R.O. Office visits to general surgeons: National ambulatory medical care survey: United States, 1975. Advance Data, Vital and Health Statistics of the National Center for Health Statistics, U.S. DHEW, No. 23, March 24, 1978.

9. Gagnon, R.O. Office visits by persons aged 65 and over: National ambulatory medical care survey: United States, 1975. Advance Data, Vital and Health Statistics of the National Center of Health Statistics, U.S. DHEW, No. 22, March 22, 1978.

10. Hing, E., Zapollo, A.: A Comparison of Nursing Home Residents and Discharges from the 1977 National Nursing Home Survey: United States. Advance Data, Vital and Health Statistics of the National Center for Health Statistics, U.S. DHEW, No. 29, May 17, 1978.

11. Howie, I.J. Utilization of selected medical practitioners: United States, 1974. Advance Data, Vital and Health Statistics of the National Center for Health Statistics, U.S. DHEW, No. 24, 1978.

12. Koch, H., Gagnon, R.O., and Ezzati, T. 1976 summary: National ambulatory medical care survey. Advance Data, Vital and Health Statistics of the National Center for Health Statistics, U.S. DHEW, No. 30, July 13, 1978.

13. Koch, H. Office visits to cardiovascular specialists: National ambulatory medical care survey: United States, 1975. Advance Data, Vital and Health Statistics of the National Center for Health Statistics, U.S. DHEW, No. 42, October 31, 1978.

14. Koch, H. Office visits to doctors of osteopathy, National ambulatory medical care survey: United States, 1975. Advance Data, Vital and Health Statistics of the National Center for Health Statistics, U.S. DHEW, No. 24, May 22, 1978.

15. Koch, H. and Ezzati, T. Office visits to ophthalmologists: National ambulatory medical care survey: United States, 1976. Advance Data, Vital and Health Statistics of the National Center for Health Statistics, U.S. DHEW, No. 31, July 14, 1978.

16. Koch, H. Office visits to orthopedic surgeons: National ambulatory medical care survey: United States, 1975-76. Advance Data, Vital and Health Statistics of the National Center for Health Statistics, U.S. DHEW, No. 33, July 18, 1978.

17. Koch, H. Office visits to otolaryngologists: National ambulatory medical care survey: United States, 1975-76. Advance Data, Vital and Health Statistics of the National Center for Health Statistics, U.S. DHEW, No. 34, August 30, 1978.

18. Koch, H. Office visits to urologists: National ambulatory medical care survey: United States, 1975-76. Advance Data, Vital and Health Statistics of the National Center for Health Statistics, U.S. DHEW, No. 39, September 7, 1978.

19. Monroe, J.T. Functional disability of geriatric patients in a family medicine program: Implications for patient care, education, and research. *J. Fam. Pract.* 7:1159, 1978.

21

Research in Primary-Care Geriatrics

Joseph M. Holtzman, Ph.D.

The research opportunities in primary-care geriatrics can be approached in at least two ways. One could catalogue and review work accomplished to date, identifying gaps and inconsistencies and suggesting research efforts and programs designed to fill these gaps. Such an approach would rest on an understanding of both the technological capabilities and political realities and limitations that currently confront us. A more speculative approach would involve going beyond what currently is and basing a discussion of research needs on a conception of what can, may, or should be. The product of such an approach would not be a catalogue of existing research projects and results or the identification of gaps. Rather, the result would be a research agenda, a charting of directions that should be taken if certain goals and objectives are to be achieved. It is this latter course that I have adopted.

In attempting to chart directions for primary-care geriatrics research, we are initially faced with a basic conceptual problem. We must face up to the question of just precisely what constitutes primary-care geriatrics. In one sense, this is an extension of the more general problem of what constitutes primary care. This issue is not of mere academic interest since the setting of a viable research agenda rests on the determination of the content, range, and scope of the problem.

One generally accepted definition of primary care describes it as "the ordinary outpatient care provided by office-based or clinic-based practitioners who are a point for first contact and appraisal and who provide less complex and continuing care to patients" [1]. This basic definition can be expanded to encompass primary-care geriatrics through the specification of age-specific criteria. Such an expansion, however, still does not answer what constitutes primary-care geriatrics, what distinguishes it from primary-care medicine and from secondary and tertiary care.

As Mechanic has pointed out, much of the discussion of what constitutes primary care (and by extension what constitutes primary-care geriatrics), confuses organizational, service, and manpower dimensions [1]. This is precisely the problem that confronts those of us who concern ourselves with research in the area. Primary care is most generally considered the province of physician generalists. Under this heading may be included general practitioners, family practitioners, general internists, and pediatricians. Excluding pediatricians from consideration, we are faced with the question of the relative competence, interest, and willingness of physician generalists to provide basic geriatric care for older individuals.

If we approach the issue of what constitutes basic geriatric care from the manpower perspective, then we are faced with a tautological definition of geriatric primary care that approximates the following: primary-care geriatrics is the care that is delivered to older patients by primary-care physicians. Such a definition suggests a research agenda that would focus on the type, amount, quality, and nature of geriatric care provided by primary-care practitioners. Such a research program might focus on the boundaries between these practitioners and secondary and tertiary care practitioners and also the boundaries among these practitioners themselves. This research would tend to be descriptive in nature and particularly useful for the documentation of what is, not for the explication of what may be. This is not to say that such research should not be undertaken. We certainly need to know who is providing the bulk of care to older individuals at this time. I would hasten to add that researchers who limit their definitions of primary care to the care delivered by the three medical specialties already mentioned will certainly be missing a large segment of the care provided by pharmacists, nurse practitioners, podiatrists, optometrists, and other limited practitioners, as well as the care provided by such marginal practitioners as chiropractors, faith healers, and others. Clearly, while the latter practitioners are not part of the health-care mainstream, it is evident that they are frequented by older individuals.

One assumption that many policy makers and researchers make is that primary-care providers are different from secondary and tertiary care providers, not only in terms of what they do but in how they do it. Their approach is thought to be holistic and person-oriented in ideal terms rather than disease oriented. Particularly in the case of family physicians, the impact of illness on the whole of the family system is said to be considered. Yet, we have no useful data to suggest that primary-care providers are significantly different in their approach to older people than other providers. Further, although social psychologists and sociologists have begun to study the impact of illness of one family member on others, we have not yet begun to address the meaning of their findings for the practitioners of clinical medicine. Research in primary care geriatrics must, in part, focus on the family system as well as the system or network of friends, neighbors, and acquaintances who are both sources of support in times of crises and useful participants in therapeutic regimens for older patients. Again, while some work in this area has begun, the potential of this network in support of efforts of primary-care physicians has been neglected.

While no fully satisfactory descriptive data on the quality of interactions between primary-care health personnel and older patients has appeared, there is little to indicate that the attitudes, willingness to serve older patients, and ability to serve these patients is much different from other providers of health and social services. For example, only one recent study has specifically explored the relationship between specialty preference, attitudes toward the aging and levels of cognitive knowledge [2]. Though the researchers found somewhat more positive attitudes toward the elderly among primary-care-oriented students than those attracted to other specialties, the findings are limited due to the nature and size of the population studied. Studies designed to identify those most willing and competent to serve the aged must be undertaken, perhaps with an eye toward guiding these individuals toward primary-care careers.

Although we have only limited knowledge regarding the practices of primary care physicians vis-a-vis the aged and know practically nothing about their level of expertise in the care of the older patient, movement has begun for the inclusion of training in geriatrics as a regular part of undergraduate medical education on the assumption that medical student education is deficient in this area. Certainly, researchers have documented relatively negative attitudes regarding the aged among medical students [3]. But little is known about how these attitudes are formed and why they persist. Even less is known about the relationship between attitudes, levels of cognitive knowledge, and actual practices. Although numerous curricular designs and modifications have been proposed in the hope of modifying student attitudes, levels of knowledge, and behaviors, their impact will be difficult to assess in light of the absence of adequate baseline data. Clearly, a major longitudinal study must be undertaken in order to determine where and how modifications in the medical curriculum might be made in order to improve the education of medical students and, ultimately, the care received by older patients.

Little is currently known about the competence of practicing primary-care personnel to deal with the special problems of the aged. It has been almost a decade since Coe and Brehm [4] produced their large-scale study of the practicing physician's ability to distinguish normal aging processes from pathological states. Although additional small-scale studies have been undertaken [5], we still have no clear picture of the practicing health-care professional's conception of normality as it relates to older patients. We have no reliable data whatever for use in determining the types and quality of care provided by nonphysician or nurse providers in primary-care settings. Clearly, a need exists for a comprehensive study of the nature, type, and outcomes of the encounters of primary-care providers with older patients. An attempt must be made to specify, quantify, and evaluate what constitutes the care provided by primary-care practitioners and what distinguishes this care from services provided by other components of the health-care system.

Thus far, we have been focusing on manpower and training issues. Closely tied to these questions is the need to evaluate alternative models of what could be. In part, these are organizational issues but to a larger extent they are policy issues. For example, reasonably good data exist that describe the patterns of health services utilization by older persons; yet, little is known regarding the persistence of these patterns over time. Only recently, work has appeared that focuses on the long-term consistency of utilization behaviors [6]. We are beginning to learn what the preferences of older individuals are in regard to how their care is organized [7]; yet, we know little in regard to which organizational arrangements produce the highest quality care for older people. Can primary-care physicians meet most of the health-care needs of older patients? Could nurse practitioners, physicians' assistants, and various paraprofessional practitioners be used to advantage? In what settings can care be most effectively provided? Should we stress home, office, clinic-based, or institutional care? How do we balance efficiency, cost, and patient preferences? Each of these questions has objective and subjective components and each needs to be addressed systematically through carefully thought out and executed research.

Allow me to propose a minimal research agenda for those working in the field of primary-care geriatrics. This agenda is minimal in the sense that it is limited in scope and in range to the most essential problems and questions that we must begin to answer if we are to plan and provide intelligently for the care of older patients. Further, I have limited this discussion to behavioral, organizational, training, and policy questions since it is these spheres that most directly influence primary-care providers and patients.

As indicated previously, useful data regarding the illness behavior of older persons have only recently emerged. While we have had statistical data available for some time that describe the utilization behavior of older people (number of episodes of hospitalization, length of stay, mean number of physician visits per year, and so on), we know very little about what prompts older people to seek out health services. How do they interpret signs and symptoms of disease, what are their health beliefs, what role do family members, friends, and acquaintances play in encouraging or discouraging them from seeking help? How well do they comply with various therapeutic regimens? What barriers prevent them from seeking help? How satisfied are they with care they receive from primary-care physicians? These are all questions that are yet to be adequately answered and that are directly related to the types, settings, levels, and quality of care sought out and provided.

Parallel research programs need to be undertaken in the area of provider behavior. In order to make intelligent decisions regarding manpower, we need to understand the behavior of health providers who care for older individuals. What factors influence provider willingness to serve older patients? What sorts of referral patterns currently exist or should be encouraged? How do physicians make decisions regarding therapeutic regimens for older patients? To what extent do the acceptance of negative stereotypes and myths about aging and the lack of training affect clinical practice? What territorial boundaries exist among the existing specialties in regard to the provision of care to older people? What territorial disputes are likely to emerge and how are these disputes likely to influence the nature and type of care available? What types of training will be necessary to meet the projected health-care needs of an aging population?

The implications of various organizational formats for the delivery of health services to older individuals has been one of the most neglected areas of research. It is also potentially one of the most important. Frequently, our thinking regarding possible formats has been constrained by current structural patterns and traditional arrangements. Clearly, a need exists to free our thinking of these constraints and to test the efficiency, acceptability, and quality of nontraditional settings and arrangements for the delivery of primary-care health services to older individuals. Model programs that provide for the formal coordination and integration of primary, secondary, and tertiary care services need to be developed, tested, and evaluated. The preferences of patients as well as providers must be established and considered. While some evidence already exists that arrangements, such as home care, geriatric day care, and geriatric foster care, have their place in the comprehensive supportive network, further creative work must be done and their utility, costs, and effectiveness established.

Finally, we must begin to think systematically about the concrete implications of federal and state policy regarding primary-care geriatrics. Decisions are being made at both of these levels that will influence the content of care and the context within which it will be delivered to older patients. The National Institute on Aging has already proclaimed a policy of discouraging the emergence of geriatrics as a specialty in the United States while the State of Ohio has, by administrative fiat, required its state supported medical schools to develop an office or department of geriatrics. These actions have been taken on the basis of only the limited available information without apparent in-depth analysis of implications of such actions. Researchers concerned with the shape of geriatric care in coming years need to begin to spell out for policy makers the likely outcomes of their actions and to do so not only on the basis of speculation but through creative, comparative, cross-national, and historic research. Without the undertaking of this necessary research, we will continue to operate blindly, to make decisions, based not on facts, but on suppositions.

Key research areas and some preliminary questions that must be addressed have been presented. No attempt to propose limits has been made but rather efforts to spell out broad avenues have been explored. What I hope I have communicated is both a sense of excitement for the possible and a sense of urgency regarding the need to begin.

References

1. Mechanic, D. *Medical Sociology: A Comprehensive Text*. New York: The Free Press, 1978.

2. Holtzman, J.M., Toewe, C.H., and Beck, J.D. Specialty preference and attitudes toward the aged. *J. Fam. Prac.* 9(4):667, 1979.

3. Holtzman, J.M., Beck, J.D., and Ettinger, R.L. Cognitive knowledge and

attitudes toward the aged of dental and medical students. Educational Gerontology: An International Quarterly (in press).

4. Coe, R. and Brehm, H. *Preventive Health Care for Adults.* New Haven: College and University Press, 1972.

5. Dye, C. and Sassenroth, D. Identification of normal aging and disease-related processes by health care professionals. *J. Am. Geriatrics Soc.* 27(10): 472, 1979.

6. Havens, B. and Mossey, J. Health care use behaviors among the elderly. Paper presented at the 32nd Annual Meeting of the Gerontological Society, Washington, D.C., November, 1979.

7. Auerbach, M.I., Gordon, D.W., Ullmann, A. and Weisel, M.J. Health care in a selected urban elderly population: Utilization patterns and perceived need. *Gerontologist* 17(4):341, 1977.

IV Research

22 Introduction

John W. Rowe, M.D.

There is, at long last, a sense of optimism among those who have long been committed to the development of geriatric medicine. The last several years have witnessed a dramatic increase in educational activities in geriatric medicine in American medical schools. Clinical and preclinical courses in gerontology and geriatrics are now available in many schools and postgraduate geriatric training programs are being developed.

I believe this optimism may be premature. Many of the current educational programs lack a strong academic underpinning and, unless such a foundation is developed, these efforts in geriatrics may be short lived or substantially reduced. Much of the present success relates to the overwhelming demographic imperative and the honeymoon effect of being a newly recognized area of importance. This advantage must be used to rapidly establish broad-based, formal, permanent programs in aging.

Despite the recent interest in geriatric medicine at medical schools, the subject is at or near the bottom of the "prestige ladder" in academic medicine. Among preclinical faculty, gerontology is often viewed as a "soft" area with little credibility. Among the clinical faculty, we have strong allies in general internal medicine, primary care, family practice, neurology, psychiatry, and rehabilitative medicine. Outside of these areas, our efforts find little support in most American medical schools. This state of affairs is a result of the newness of our efforts, the lack of awareness of most medical school faculty members of the data base of gerontology and geriatrics, and the fact that geriatric medicine has generally developed as a clinical activity without a research base.

While we should not strive toward a more "prestigious" position among our fellow faculty members just for the sake of our own self image, American academic geriatrics must develop into a much more credible area of activity if our educational programs are to survive. Persistence of present attitudes among faculty will result in failure of academic geriatricians and gerontologists to be promoted, discontinuation of the access to curriculum that we have recently achieved, and shunting of educational activities in geriatrics to a subset of one or several relevant clinical departments.

The establishment, on the other hand, of a productive, sophisticated research program, whether it be basic science or clinical geriatrics, will serve several useful goals. We are clearly skating on thin ice in geriatric medicine with regard to our data base. Research is very badly needed in order to firm up and expand our knowledge of health and disease in old age and to stimulate continued growth of educational programs. In addition, research programs will provide a permanent, formal home for academic faculty whose major interest is in aging, and research funding will in all likelihood subsidize the teaching efforts of such faculty as has been true in other fields. Establishment of productive, peer-reviewed, research programs will provide stability for activities in aging, establish a career ladder in academic geriatric medicine, enhance our access to curriculum time as well as to resources at the medical school, and increase our capacity to attract students and adequate numbers of new faculty.

The next decade will be a crucial time for American academic geriatrics. We may emerge from the 1980s as a unified, broad-based, multidisciplinary enterprise with a sizable cadre of academically trained and academically oriented gerontologists and geriatricians. On the other hand, if we fail to establish our proper position, we will remain a loose-knit group of faculty based in several departments, joined by a common interest but with little clout in academe, and our educational efforts will suffer accordingly.

The success or failure of our efforts to establish aging as an independent activity in medical schools will be reflected in the structure of developing postgraduate training programs. If aging survives academically in American medicine, then core fellowship programs in gerontology and geriatrics will flourish. In these programs, individuals will train for two to three years in various clinical aspects of geriatric medicine as well as the biomedical data base of geriatrics and will gain research and teaching experience. Trainees in such programs will populate academic programs in geriatric medicine and become the trainers of the next generation of medical students. If it does not survive as a separate entity, then it is likely that postgraduate training programs in geriatric medicine will become a special "track" in training programs in general internal medicine, primary care and family practice. One-year focused programs in geriatrics will be available to specialists in certain relevant areas, such as psychiatry and neurology, who wish to broaden their base and expertise in this area. Graduates of such training programs, while certainly capable of participating in geriatric education programs at the medical-school level, would lack the broad geriatric and gerontologic base needed to develop multidisciplinary academic programs involving basic science as well as clinical activities.

We are at a crossroads in geriatric medicine, and developments over the next decade will determine the ultimate scope and quality of our educational activities. The development over this time of integrated, broad-based, productive, research programs in the preclinical and clinical areas will be the vital link in the establishment of permanent, formal programs in aging at American medical schools.

23

Evidence for an Age-Related Increase in Sympathetic Nervous System Activity

John W. Rowe, M.D.

Interest in a possible relation between aging and the sympathoadrenal system has recently been fostered by the availability of reliable techniques for the measurement of catecholamines in plasma and increasing knowledge of their physiologic effects. This chapter will briefly review current information regarding the influence of age on the function of the sympathetic nervous system in man. For a more detailed treatment the reader is referred to a recent review [1].

Basal Determinations: Methodological Considerations

Presently, available information regarding the influence of age on basal circulating norepinephrine levels is conflicting and perhaps can best be evaluated in light of the varying definition of "basal" used by different investigators. In this regard, particular attention should be paid to three variables: posture, feeding, and time of day.

Upright posture is universally recognized as a stimulus for sympathetic activity, and all studies have been performed with the subjects supine before study. However, the length of time individuals were supine before blood samples were drawn varies from 10 min to 8 h. The potential importance of this has recently been stressed by Saar and Gordon [2], who evaluated the influence of length of time recumbent on plasma norepinephrine in young and old individuals. Thirty minutes after recumbency, plasma catecholamines (norepinephrine plus epinephrine) were higher in the elderly individual than in the young (3.66 ± 0.54 vs 1.66 ± 1.19 pmol/ml; $P < 0.01$). After 9 hours of recumbency, however, catecholamine levels had fallen in both groups and were no longer significantly different (old, 1.79 ± 0.33 pmol/ml; young, 1.47 ± 0.15 pmol/ml). In a subsequent larger series, whereas plasma catecholamines fell during 9 hours of recumbency in both young and old, the old group maintained a borderline significantly higher level than the young group.

Another consideration in the definition of basal activity relates to feeding and fasting. Since feeding has now been shown to increase sympathetic activity in animals and human beings [3], consideration of samples drawn during the postprandial period as being "basal" must now be judged questionable.

A third consideration in evaluation of "basal" data relates to the time of day of sample collection. Prinz et al. [4] have shown that plasma norepinephrine levels fall throughout the day with a peak level in the morning and the lowest level during a sleep between 2300 and 0900 h in both young and old individuals. This is particularly relevant to the present discussion since, in several investigations that compared plasma norepinephrine levels in the young and old, blood samples were collected at varying times throughout the day and can include an effect of this circadian variation in catecholamines.

Basal Circulating Norepinephrine Levels

Over a dozen papers have now appeared in the literature that report basal circulating norepinephrine levels in men and women of varying age. Despite the uncertainty introduced by the varying definition of basal, the general impression from presently available information is that there is an increase in basal circulating norepinephrine with advancing age. In an early report utilizing modern assay techniques, Christensen [5] reported in 1973 that plasma norepinephrine rose approximately 2-fold from 200 pg/ml to 400 pg/ml between ages 20 and 70 in 16 healthy individuals aged 27 to 77. These individuals were all fasting and supine overnight. This initial report was confirmed by a 1975 study by Pedersen and Christensen [6], who found plasma norepinephrine to rise with age in a group of 32 nonhypertensive controls aged 20 to 65. In this study, individuals were fasting overnight but were supine only for 30 min. In a series of papers, Ziegler, Lake, Palmer, Kopin, and Coleman [7-10] found plasma norepinephrine levels to rise with advancing age. In these studies, subjects were not fasting, samples were obtained at various times between 0800 and 1600 h, and subjects were supine for at least 20 min. In their first report in 1976, Ziegler et al. [9] found a significant positive correlation between basal plasma norepinephrine levels and age in 38 individuals aged 10 to 65. This report was confirmed by Lake et al. [8], who reported a larger series from the same laboratory of 74 individuals aged 10 to 70. In this report, mean levels rose from approximately 230 pg/ml at age 20 to approximately 380 pg/ml at age 70.

In 1977, these same investigators [9] compared the plasma norepinephrine level in normotensive and hypertensive individuals from across the adult age range. They again found that in 84 normal individuals aged 15 to 63, plasma norepinephrine rose with age and that these levels were not different from those found in hypertensive subjects, suggesting that the previously reported increase in norepinephrine with essential hypertension may have been related to the greater age of the hypertensive than the normal subjects studied. In the most recent report from this laboratory, Palmer et al. [11] found that basal plasma norepinephrine levels were higher in a group of 14 old men (mean age, 53 ± 0.8 yr) than in a group of seven young subjects (mean age, 14 ± 0.9 yr). Two reports by Coulombe et al. [11,12], using a less-sensitive fluorometric method for measurement of plasma norepinephrine, also indicate a highly significant increase in basal norepinephrine levels in fasting individuals who were supine for 15 min. Other reports indicating higher basal plasma norepinephrine levels in old individuals than young individuals include those of Franco-Morselli et al. [13] (11 subjects aged 20 to 76); Sever et al. [14] (35 subjects aged 36 to 64); and Prinz et al. [4] (9 young, aged 21 to 28 and 5 old, aged 62 to 80). In contrast, in a recent report Young et al. [16] failed to detect an effect of age on basal plasma norepinephrine levels when comparing a group of healthy young (15 subjects aged 18 to 33) and old (12 subjects aged 67 to 83) individuals. In this study, all individuals were supine and fasting overnight.

It seems certain at the present time that there is no decrease in basal circulating norepinephrine with age and that it is likely but not proven that there is an increase. The physiological significance of such an increase, if present, might relate to several age-related physiological changes, including decreased end-organ responsiveness or central nervous system changes resulting in less-tonic inhibitory input into the brain-stem areas regulating sympathetic outflow.

Sympathetic Nervous System Responsiveness to Hemodynamic Stimuli

Although there are only a few published reports comparing plasma norepinephrine response to hemodynamic stimulation in young and old individuals, the bulk of the available data indicates an age-related increase in sympathetic responsivity. In 1976, Ziegler and coworkers [7] reported that plasma norepinephrine response to upright posture after 20 min supine and to isometric exercise increased linearly with age. More recently, Young et al. [16] reported that the increase in plasma norepinephrine while standing was greater in healthy old individuals than in healthy young individuals, despite similar changes in blood pressure and pulse. Of particular interest in this same study was the finding that plasma norepinephrine persisted at significantly higher levels in the old subjects than in the young subjects 15 min after return to recumbency. Since these same investigators have reported no effect of age on the disappearance of norepinephrine from plasma, with a plasma half-time of disappearance of 1.9 to 2.0 min in young and old individuals [16], the persistence of this high level 15 min after recumbency suggests that the sympathetic responsivity is not only greater in old individuals but more sustained.

These findings, however, are in accord with the previously noted observation by Saar and Gordon [2] that the differential between young and old individuals in plasma norepinephrine that is present 30 min after recumbency is diminished or absent after prolonged recumbency. Palmer et al. [10] studied the plasma norepinephrine response to upright posture followed by an isometric exercise (handgrip) and cold pressor test in young and old individuals. In this study, basal norepinephrine levels were higher in the old group than in the young, and both groups exhibited equivalent increases in norepinephrine above basal after 5 min standing. The addition of the isometric exercise to the posture stimulus resulted in greater additional increase in norepinephrine in the old group than in the young. In the cold pressor test, plasma norepinephrine levels were obtained in 5 young and 3 old subjects before and after the test. Despite the small number of subjects, the old individuals had significantly higher basal norepinephrine levels than the young group. Plasma norepinephrine rose after the cold pressor test in both groups. The increase above basal in the older subjects was greater, though not significantly so in this small study, than the increase above basal in the young group. In studies in which basal and post-standing plasma norepinephrine levels were obtained in hypertensive subjects and age-matched normotensive controls, Franco-Morselli et al. [13] and Sever et al. [14] both reported that the increase in plasma norepinephrine above basal with upright posture increases with age.

Possible Mechanism Underlying Age-Related Increase in Sympathetic Responsiveness to Hemodynamic Stimuli

Baroreceptor reflexes play a major role in blood pressure regulation via tonic regulation of the activity of the vasomotor center. Baroreceptors are mechano-receptors, and when they are stimulated by stretching of the vessel wall, as occurs in hypertension, increased baroreceptor nerve activity and inhibition of the vasomotor center occurs. This results in a decreased central sympathetic nervous system outflow acting to return arterial pressure to normal and decrease stretch in the baroreceptor.

Responsivity of the baroreceptor reflex has been shown to decrease with age in man. Cribbin et al. [17] evaluated the change in heart rate after phenyle-phrine-induced increases in blood pressure in young and old individuals and found a significant effect of age on the magnitude of the heart rate reduction for any given increase in blood pressure. The age-related changes in baroreceptor sensitivity suggest a possible mechanism for the age-related increase in responsi-bility of the sympathetic nervous system to hemodynamic stimuli (figure 23-1). It is established that stiffening of the carotid artery in experimental settings results in resetting of the sensitivity of the baroreceptor [18]. Such a resetting is reflected in decreased impulse traffic in the carotid sinus nerve for any given blood pressure level compared to nonhypertensive controls. The decreased sensi-tivity of the baroreceptor in the elderly can be due to the well-known decrease in arterial distensibility associated with age. This would result in less tonic inhi-bition of the vasomotor center. That stiffening results in hypertension is well known and consistent in our view with an increased basal blood pressure seen in the elderly [19]. A sensitized vasomotor center would result in greater basal central sympathetic outflow and might account for an age-related increase in

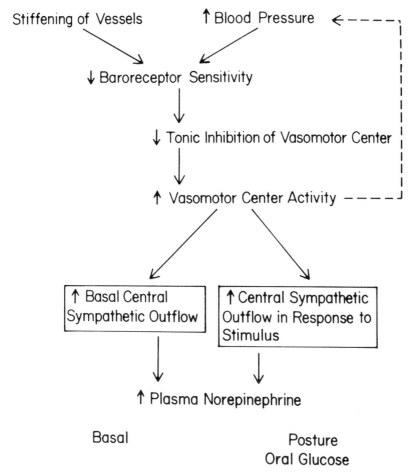

Figure 23-1. Schema for possible mechanism whereby age-related stiffening of carotid artery would lead to increased sympathetic nervous system activity. Reproduced with permission from Rowe, J.W. and Troen B.R. *Endocrine Reviews* 1:167, 1980.

basal plasma norepinephrine and the enhance response of the elderly to hemo-dynamic stimulation.

Conclusion

Consideration of the presently available literature regarding human aging and sympathetic nervous system activity permits development of the view that old age may represent a hyperadrenergic state. In posture studies, not only is the peak plasma norepinephrine level greater in old than in young subjects, but also, when studied, the increase has been found to be more sustained in the elderly than in the young. Since normal daily activities are punctuated by frequent stimuli for sympathetic nervous system activation, such an attainment of upright posture, feeding, exercise, and psychological stress or excitement, it is possible that a prolonged or more sustained response in the elderly than in young individuals to these frequent stimuli would induce a constant hyperadrenergic state in the elderly under "normal" circumstances. Such a state might have physiological consequences not only in the area of carbohydrate tolerance, but also in several other clearly age-related physiological changes, such as fragmented sleep, cognitive impairment, and hypertension.

References

1. Rowe, J.W. and Troen, B.R. Sympathetic nervous system and aging in man. *Endocrine Reviews* 1(2):167, 1980.

2. Saar, N. and Gordon, R.D. Variability of plasma catecholamine levels: age, duration of posture and time of day. *Br. J. Clin. Pharmacol.* 8:353, 1979.

3. Young, J.B. and Landsberg, L. Suppression of sympathetic nervous system during fasting. *Science* 196:1473, 1977.

4. Prinz, P.N., Halter, J., Benedetti, C., and Raskind, M. Circadian variation of plasma catecholamines in young and old men: relation to rapid eye movement and slow wave sleep. *J. Clin. Endocrinol. Metab.* 49:300, 1979.

5. Christensen, N.J. Plasma noradrenaline and adrenaline in patients with thyrotoxicosis and myxoedema. *Clin. Sci. Mol. Med.* 45:163, 1973.

6. Pedersen, E.B. and Christensen, N.H. Catecholamines in plasma and urine in patients with essential hypertension determined by double-isotope derivative techniques. *Acta. Med. Scand.* 198:373, 1975.

7. Ziegler, M.G., Lake, C.R., and Kopin, I.J. Plasma noradrenaline increases with age. *Nature* 261:333, 1976.

8. Lake, C.R., Ziegler, M.G., and Kopin, I.J. Use of plasma norepinephrine for evaluation of sympathetic neuronal function in man. *Life Sci.* 18:1315, 1976.

9. Lake, C.R., Ziegler, M.G., Coleman, M.D., and Kopin, I.J. Age-adjusted plasma norepinephrine levels are similar in normotensive and hypertensive subjects. *N. Engl. J. Med.* 296:208, 1977.

10. Palmer, G.J., Ziegler, M.G. and Lake, C.R. Response of norepinephrine and blood pressure to stress increases with age. *J. Gerontol.* 33:482, 1978.

11. Coulombe, P., Dussault, J.H. and Walker, P. Plasma catecholamine concentrations in hyperthyroidism and hypothyroidism. *Metabolism* 25:973, 1976.

12. Coulombe, P., Dussault, J.H., and Walker, P. Catecholamine metabolism in thyroid disease. II. Norepinephrine secretion rate in hyperthyroidism and hypothyroidism. *J. Clin. Endocrinol. Metab.* 44:185, 1977.

13. Franco-Morselli, R., Elghozi, J.L., Joly, E., DiGiuilio, S., and Meyer, P. Increased plasma adrenaline concentrations in benign essential hypertension. *Br. Med. J.* 2:1251, 1977.

14. Sever, P.S., Osikowska, B., Birch, M., and Tunbridge, R.D.G. Plasma noradrenaline in essential hypertension. *Lancet* 1:1078, 1977.

15. DeChamplain, J., and Cousineau, D. Lack of correlation between age and circulating catecholamines in hypertensive patients. *N. Engl. J. Med.* 297: 672, 1977.

16. Young, J.R., Rowe, J.W., Pallotta, J.A., Sparrow, D., and Landsberg, L. Enhanced plasma norepinephrine response to upright posture and oral glucose administration in elderly human subjects. *Metabolism* 29:498, 1980.

17. Cribbin, B., Pickering, T.G., Sleight, P., and Peto, R. Effect of age and high blood pressure on baroreflex sensitivity in man. *Cir. Res.* 29:424, 1971.

18. McCubbin, J.W., and Ferrario, C.N., Baroreceptor reflexes and hypertension. In J. Genest, E. Koiw, and O. Kurchel (Eds) *Hypertension.* New York: McGraw-Hill, 1977.

19. Kohn, R.R. Heart and cardiovascular system. In C.E. Finch and L. Hayflick (Eds) *1977 Handbook of the Biology of Aging.* New York: Van Nostrand Reinhold, 1977.

24 Drug Metabolism and Therapeutics in the Elderly

Robert E. Vestal, M.D.

With the recognition that the aged constitute an increasing proportion of our patient population, attention is being directed toward understanding the epidemiology, pharmacology and toxicology of drug use in the elderly. In addition to discussing pertinent epidemiological considerations, this chapter summarizes some of the physiological differences associated with aging and illustrates how they can lead to age difference in drug disposition and drug response. Practical aspects of geriatric therapeutics are also included. The reader wishing a more detailed treatment of this subject is encouraged to consult several comprehensive reviews [1,2,3].

During the last decade, geriatric clinical pharmacology, has become the focus of considerable research activity. Prior to 1971, there were few studies published and most were poorly designed or anecdotal. This situation has changed dramatically, and we are seeing a proliferation of scientific reports, books, and published symposia. Recognizing the importance of this area, the National Institute on Aging has identified pharmacology as having high priority for research. Some limitations should be kept in mind, however. Although statistically valid age differences or correlations with age can be demonstrated, biological variation can preclude clinically useful generalizations regarding the effects of age [4]. The elderly in many ways are a more heterogeneous group than the young. It should also be emphasized that all currently available studies are cross-sectional rather than longitudinal in design. As such, they can only provide information about differences rather than changes with age. This distinction is important for the gerontologist because age differences in cross-sectional studies do not necessarily reflect the intrinsic biological effects of aging. For example, environmental changes with time can lead to cohort differences due to selective mortality, which, in the strict sense, are separate from the effects of aging per se [5].

Epidemiological Aspects of Drug Use in the Elderly

The elderly constitute a growing segment of the American people. The aged now spend almost $3 billion (about 25% of the national total) for drugs and drug

This research was supported in part by the Medical Research Service of the Veterans Administration.

sundries. If current trends continue through the next 50 years, expenditures by the elderly for drugs can reach 40% of the national total. Although the average annual expenditure is just over $100 per capita, the figure is more than three-fold higher for nursing home patients, who take on the average more than four different drugs per day. Some segments of our health-care delivery system bear a disproportionate burden of the health care needs of the aged. Thus, the Veterans Administration anticipates that between 1970 and 2000 adult males aged 65 or older who are veterans will increase from 26% to 59%. These demographic considerations emphasize that the needs of geriatric patients will constitute an increasingly important aspect of medical care for the future.

Older patients have a roughly two-fold greater incidence of adverse reactions to drugs than younger patients [6]. This is not particularly surprising. Elderly patients have multiple diseases, which often require multiple drugs. Since the incidence of adverse drug reactions increases with the number of drugs administered, the elderly are predisposed to complications arising from the drug use. In addition, errors in comprehension and compliance are common. One study in an outpatient setting found that 59% of patients aged 60 or older made one or more medication errors and 26% made potentially serious errors [7]. The average number of errors was 2.6 errors per patient. The most frequent error was omission of medication, followed by lack of knowledge about medications, use of medications not prescribed by the physician, and errors of dosage, sequence, or timing. Finally, disease-related alterations in physiology can affect both drug metabolism and drug response.

Physiological Aspects of Geriatric Pharmacology

A number of factors that might be expected to affect drug disposition and response in the elderly are listed in table 24-1. Elevated gastric pH, delayed gastric emptying, reduced intestinal blood flow as well as other age-related alterations in gastrointestinal physiology could affect drug absorption after oral administration. The available data are limited but do not indicate a significant alteration of absorption in the elderly.

By contrast drug distribution has been shown to be affected by age. Body composition is an important determinant of drug distribution and differs with age. Total body water, both in absolute terms and as a percentage of body weight, has been shown to decline by 10% to 15% between the ages of 20 and 90. Lean body mass in proportion to body weight also is diminished and seems to be due to a relative increase of 10% to 20% in body fat with age. Drugs that are distributed mainly in body water or lean body mass might have higher blood levels, particularly if the dose is based on total body weight or surface area. Ethanol, for example, distributes in body water, and higher peak ethanol levels were observed in older subjects without a difference in rates of metabolism [8].

Table 24-1

Summary of Factors Affecting Drug Disposition and Response in the Elderly

Effect	Altered Physiology	Clinical Importance
Absorption	Elevated gastric pH Reduced GI blood flow ? Reduced number of absorbing cells ? Reduced GI motility	Not sufficiently studied

Distribution	Body composition
	Reduced total
	    body water
	Reduced lean body
	    mass/kg body weight
	Increased body fat
		Higher concentration of drugs dis-
		    tributed in body fluids
		? Longer duration of action of fat
		    soluble drugs

	Protein binding Reduced serum albumin	Higher free fraction of highly protein bound drugs

Elimination	Hepatic metabolism
	Reduced enzyme activity
	Reduced hepatic mass
	Reduced hepatic blood flow
		Apparently slower biotransformation
		    of some drugs
		Influenced by environmental factors
		    (e.g. nutrition and smoking)

	Renal excretion Reduced glomerular filtra- tion rate Reduced renal plasma flow Altered tubular function	Slower excretion of some drugs
Response	Multiple disease states Multiple drug use common Altered receptor sensitivity Organ specific age differences	More variation in dose response Adverse drug reactions

From Vestal, 1978.

The age-dependent increase in the volume of distribution for diazepam, a very lipid-soluble drug found by Klotz et al. [9], could be due to an increase in body fat.

Many drugs are bound to albumin in the plasma. The reduction in serum albumin concentration with age means fewer available binding sites. For example, Miller et al. [10] reported an 11% decrease in serum albumin concentration and a 25% increase in the unbound fraction of tolbutamide in an older group of healthy subjects compared to a younger group (table 24-2). Since more unbound drug would be available for distribution and metabolism, it was suggested that age differences in the pharmacokinetics of tolbutamide might be found. This may be the case for phenytoin. In one study [11], total plasma clearance was negatively correlated with serum albumin and was greater in old than young subjects (figure 24-1). Thus, age differences in plasma binding have been found for some drugs studied, but not all (table 24-3). Unfortunately, the

Table 24-2

Effect of Age on Protein and Albumin Concentrations and Unbound Fraction of Tolbutamide[a]

	Young Group (N=24)	Old Group (N=19)
Age (yr)	38.74 ± 10.76	72.05 ± 8.50
Weight (kg)	79.37 ± 2.14	74.25 ± 1.91[b]
Serum protein concentration (g/100 ml)	7.25 ± 0.11	7.22 ± 0.51
Serum albumin concentration (g/100 ml)	5.25 ± 0.54	4.67 ± 0.65[b]
Unbound fraction of tolbutamide[c]	0.032 ± 0.006	0.040 ± 0.007[d]

From Miller et al., 1978.
[a] Mean ± standard deviation.
[b] Significantly different (p < 0.01; t-test).
[c] Total plasma tolbutamide concentration of 100 µg/ml.
[d] Significantly different (p < 0.001; t-test).

Table 24-3

Effect of Age on Protein Binding of Drugs in Young and Old Subjects

Age Difference Found	No Age Difference Found
Chlormethiazole	Chlordiazepoxide
Lorazepam	Desmethyldiazepam
Meperidine*	Diazepam
Phenylbutazone	Meperidine*
Phenytoin*	Oxazepam
Tolbutamide	Penicillin G
Warfarin*	Phenobarbituric Acid
	Phenytoin*
	Quinidine
	Salicylate
	Sulfadiazine
	Warfarin*

Source: Vestal, R.E. Aging and pharmacokinetics: Impact of altered physiology in the elderly. In A. Cherkin, C.E. Finch, N. Karash, T. Makinodan, F.L. Scott, and B. Strehler (Eds.) *Physiology and Cell Biology of Aging.* Vol. 9. New York: Raven Press, 1979.
*Different studies report conflicting results for the same drug.

results of some studies are conflicting, possibly due to differences in subject selection and the techniques used.

Removal of drugs from the body occurs principally by two routes: (1) liver metabolism to less active or inactive metabolites, which are usually excreted by the kidney, or (2) excretion of unchanged drug by the kidney. Both of these processes may be altered in the elderly.

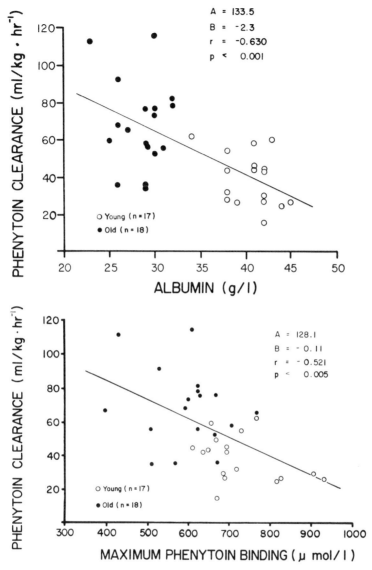

Figure 24-1. Correlations of phenytoin clearance with serum albumin (upper panel) and maximum phenytoin binding (lower panel). Total plasma clearance was determined in young subjects (aged 20 to 38) and old subjects (aged 65-90) after 250 mg phenytoin. Maximum plasma binding was determined from measurements of free and bound drug at four different drug concentrations. Figure based on data from Hayes et al., 1975.

Studies in experimental animals have shown reduced liver microsomal enzyme induction with aging. Although there are no similar direct studies of the effects of age on liver drug-metabolizing enzyme activity in man, it is known that liver mass and liver blood flow decline with age. There is also evidence that the aging process can result in alteration of the intrinsic capacity of the liver for the biotransformation of some drugs. Studies with antipyrine, for example, have consistently reported a prolonged half-life and reduced metabolic clearance in older subjects [4,12,13,14]. In one study, this was found even when clearance was adjusted for an estimate of liver mass [13]. However, in other studies, the age differences seemed to be mostly explained by a decreased sensitivity of the elderly to enzyme induction by environmental factors, such as cigarette smoking [4,14]. Theophylline is a clinically important drug for which a reduction of dosage in the elderly is recommended because of what appears to be an age-related decline in biotransformation by the liver [15]. In general, clearance is a better measure of intrinsic liver drug-metabolizing activity than half-life, since the latter is a function of both clearance and distribution volume. For drugs highly bound to plasma protein, the clearance of unbound drug should be determined before making conclusions about an effect of age on metabolism. Not all drugs that have been studied show an effect of age on half-life or clearance (table 24-4), and some studies conducted by different investigators with different groups of subjects, but using the same drug, have given differing results. Once again, this is probably due to differences in methodology and study population.

The decline in renal function with advancing age has been well documented. For drugs or active metabolites that are primarily excreted by the kidney, this means that clearance can be impaired in older patients and plasma levels can be higher after doses that are standard for younger patients. Several examples are listed in table 24-5. We all know that the dosage of drugs, such as the aminoglycoside antibiotics, digoxin, and lithium, needs to be reduced in the presence of renal insufficiency. However, biological variation is such that we must still use plasma levels to guide therapy with drugs that have serious toxic side effects.

Alterations in Drug Response in the Elderly

The effects of age on pharmacokinetics are of interest primarily because they may provide insight into the mechanisms of altered drug response in older patients. This area of research in geriatric clinical pharmacology has received relatively less attention than pharmacokinetics. However, several examples are available. Age has been shown to be an important variable in determining the degree of pain relief obtained following administration of a potent analgesic [16]. Under double-blind conditions, 10 mg of morphine sulfate and 20 mg of pentazocine provided an age-related increase in relief of pain intensity in 712 patients

Table 24-4
Effect of Age on the Hepatic Metabolism of Drugs in
Young and Old Subjects

Age Difference Found	No Age Difference Found
Half-Life	
Acetaminophen	Imipramine
Acetanilid	Indocyanine Green*
Aminopyrine	Indomethacin
Antipyrine	Isoniazid
Chlordiazepoxide	Lorazepam*
Chlormethiazole	Morphine
Desipramine	Nitrazepam
Diazepam	Oxazepam
Indocyanine Green*	Phenylbutazone
Lidocaine	Phenytoin
Lorazepam*	Tolbutamide
Quinidine	Warfarin
Clearance	
Acetaminophen*	Acetaminophen*
Antipyrine	Diazepam
Chlordiazepoxide	Ethanol
Chlormethiazole	Lidocaine
Indocyanine Green	Phenytoin*
Phenylbutazone	Warfarin
Phenytoin*	
Propranolol	
Quinidine	
Theophylline	
Tolbutamide	

Source: Vestal, R.E. Aging and pharmacokinetics: Impact of altered physiology in the elderly. In A. Cherkin, C.E. Finch, N. Karash, T. Makinodan, F.L. Scott, and B. Strehler (Eds.) *Physiology and Cell Biology of Aging.* Vol. 9. New York: Raven Press, 1979.
*Different studies report conflicting results for the same drug.

(figure 24-2). Available data suggest that this increased responsiveness is probably related to age differences in pain perception, rather than differences in pharmacokinetics. At least three studies have demonstrated an increased sensitivity to the effects of various benzodiazepines [17,18,19]. The elderly (figure 24-3) are more susceptible to the toxic effects of flurazepam (drowsiness, confusion, or ataxia) and for this reason a low initial dose (15 mg) is recommended [17]. By contrast, the elderly have been shown less sensitive (figure 24-4) to the chronotropic effects of isoproterenol and the beta-blocking effects of propranolol [20]. In vitro experiments using crude membrane functions from human mononuclear cells have demonstrated an age-related decline in the number of beta-adrenergic receptors without an alteration in receptor affinity [21]. Thus,

Table 24-5
Drugs Eliminated by the Kidney which have
Pharmacokinetic Age Differences

Cefradine	Lithium
Cephazolin	Penicillin G
Cimetidine	Phenobarbital
Digoxin	Practolol
Dihydrostreptomycin	Propicillin
Doxycycline	Sulphamethiazole
Kanamycin	Tetracycline

Source: Vestal, R.E. Aging and pharmacokinetics: Impact of altered physiology in the elderly. In A. Cherkin, C.E. Finch, N. Karash, T. Makinodan, F.L. Scott, and B. Strehler (Eds.) *Physiology and Cell Biology of Aging.* Vol. 9. New York: Raven Press, 1979.

while it is generally assumed that the aged will be more sensitive to drug effects, this is not necessarily the case for all drugs. In fact, the opposite may be true.

Basic Principles of Therapeutics in the Elderly

The principles of therapeutics in the elderly are essentially the same as would be applied to any patient [3].

1. *Strive for a diagnosis prior to treatment.* Symptomatic therapy may be all that can be offered, but specific therapy is usually preferable. If the patient's symptoms are due to abuse or misuse of the medications, for example, additional drug therapy is only likely to complicate the situation.

2. *Take a careful drug history.* This is especially important in the elderly, who usually will have multiple problems and be taking multiple medications. The patient may be receiving two or more drugs of the same type or with similar side effects—perhaps prescribed by the same or different clinicians. Additive anticholinergic side effects can result from concurrent use of drugs, such as antidepressants, antipsychotic agents, antihistamines, and nonprescription cold remedies. A problem-oriented medication list can be useful in this regard.

3. *Know the pharmacology of drugs prescribed.* It is better to use a few drugs well than to use many drugs poorly. Rational drug therapy is enhanced by an awareness of the route of elimination, half-life, protein-binding properties, and propensity for drug interactions, along with major pharmacological actions, side effects, and toxicity.

4. *Titrate drug dosage with patient response.* Identify signs or symptoms that can be monitored serially for effectiveness of drug therapy. Increase drug dosage gradually until the desired therapeutic end point is reached or unwanted toxicity is present or anticipated. Judicious monitoring of plasma levels can be useful.

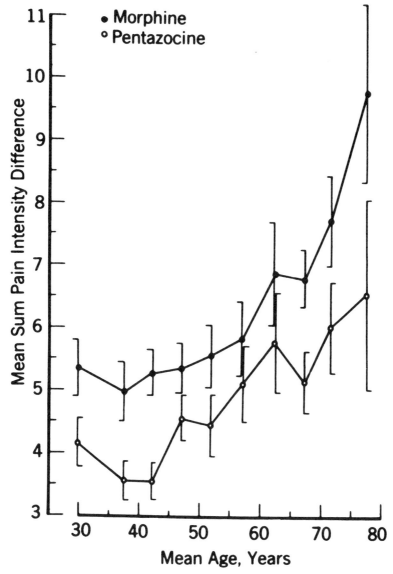

Figure 24-2. Correlation of an estimate of pain relief (mean sum pain intensity difference) with age group after 10 mg morphine (slope = 0.039, p < 0.001) and 20 mg pentazocine (slope = 0.052, p < 0.001) administered intramuscularly to 712 patients for acute postoperative pain. From Bellville, J.W. Influence of age on pain relief from analgesics. A study of postoperative patients. *JAMA* 217:1835, 1971. Reprinted with permission.

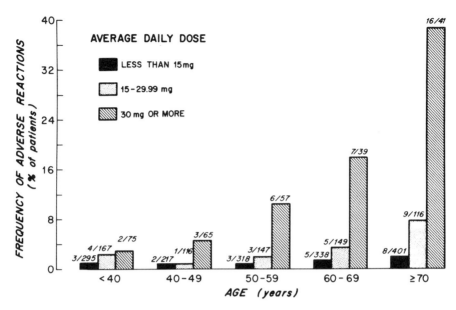

Figure 24-3. Frequency of adverse reactions to flurazepam in relation to age and average daily dose. From Greenblatt, D.J., et al. Toxicity of high-dose flurazepam in the elderly. *Clin. Pharmacol. Ther.* 21: 355, 1977. Reprinted with permission.

5. *Use smaller doses in the elderly.* The usual dose for young patients can be too large for an older patient. It is usually better to give too little drug to the older patient than to risk giving too much. Thus, caution is a virtue in geriatric therapy. While the loading dose may not require much alteration, the initial maintenance dose may need to be reduced by 25% to 50%. Examples include digoxin and theophylline.

6. *Simplify the therapeutic regimen.* Complex drug regimens can be easily mismanaged by the elderly patient with a deteriorating memory or impaired vision. In order to promote comprehension and compliance the following steps are suggested:

a. Explain the treatment plan to both the patient and a friend or relative. Give concise written instructions. Use a visiting nurse if necessary.

b. Encourage the use of a diary or calendar to record daily drug administration.

c. Choose a dosage form, perhaps an elixir, that is appropriate for the patient's physical limitations.

d. Label the drug container carefully. Specify standard containers for the patient with arthritis who cannot open safety caps.

e. Encourage the return or destruction of old unused medications. The accumu-

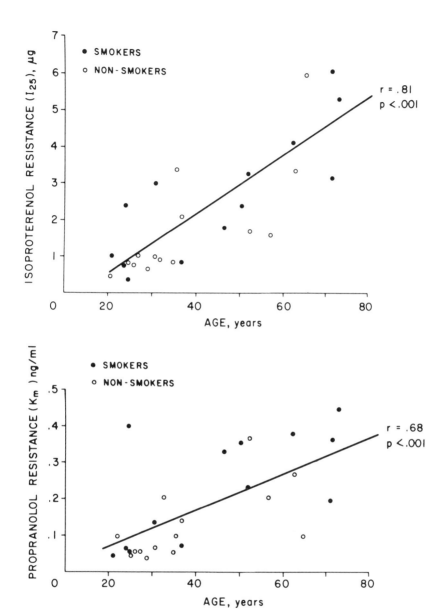

Figure 24-4. Relationship between isoproterenol resistance and age (upper panel) and between propranolol resistance and age (lower panel) in smokers (●) and nonsmokers (○). From Vestal, R.E., et al. Reduced β-adrenoceptor sensitivity in the elderly. *Clin. Pharmacol. Ther.* 26:181, 1979. Reprinted with permission.

lation of old medications from prior treatment programs will only serve to confuse the patient.

7. *Regularly review the drug regimen and discontinue those not needed.* This should be done at least every three to six months. Often drugs are continued inadvertently long after the indication for their use has disappeared.

8. *Be alert to drug-induced illness.* Drugs can be an explanation for unusual symptoms. Avoid substituting prescriptions for taking adequate medical and social histories.

Often the relationship between the clinician and the patient is more important than the drugs prescribed. Set realistic treatment goals together with the patient, and then point out clinical improvements, even if the change is small. Patients greatly appreciate having a physician who is sincerely interested in all aspects of their care, social and emotional as well as medical.

Conclusion

Altered physiology probably accounts for many of the observed age differences in drug metabolism and drug response that have been documented in the elderly. Upon this substrate of normal age differences in physiology are superimposed the pathophysiological changes associated with diseases, such as congestive heart failure, renal insufficiency and dementia, that so commonly afflict the elderly. Thus, elderly patients, the patient population who require and use the most medications, are the most at risk for adverse drug reactions.

There is a great need for additional research to further define the underlying mechanisms of aging in relation to pharmacology, to characterize age differences in pharmacokinetics and pharmacodynamics for both old and new drugs, to identify drug interactions that may be especially important in elderly patients, and to develop methods for improved drug therapy for our growing geriatric population. This is already a challenging and rewarding area of research for both basic scientists and clinical investigators interested in gerontology and geriatrics. There is also a need to incorporate our present and future understanding of geriatric clinical pharmacology into the teaching of therapeutics at all levels of medical education. Only in this way can old as well as new knowledge in this field be translated into better patient care.

References

1. Crooks, J., O'Malley, K., and Stevenson, I.H. Pharmacokinetics in the elderly. *Clin. Pharmacokinet.* 1:280, 1976.

2. Richey, D.P. and Bender, D. Pharmacokinetic consequences of aging. *Annu. Rev. Pharmacol. Toxicol.* 17:49, 1977.

3. Vestal, R.E. Drug use in the elderly: A review of problems and special considerations. *Drugs* 16:358, 1978.

4. Vestal, R.E., Norris, A.H., Tobin, J.D., Cohen, B.H., Shock, N.W., and Andres, R. Antipyrine metabolism in man: Influence of age, alcohol, caffeine, and smoking. *Clin. Pharmacol. Ther.* 18:425, 1975.

5. Rowe, J.W., Clinical research on aging: Strategies and directions. *N. Eng. J. of Med.* 297:1332, 1977.

6. Hurwitz, N. Predisposing factors in adverse reactions to drugs. *British Med. J.* 1:536, 1969.

7. Schwartz, D., Wang, M., Feitz, L., and Goss, M.E.W. Medication errors made by elderly, chronically ill patients. *Am. J. Pub. Hlth.* 52:2018, 1962.

8. Vestal P.E., Norris, A.H., Tobin, J.D., Andres, R., Norris, A.H., and Mezey, E. Aging and ethanol metabolism. *Clin. Pharmacol. Ther.* 21:343, 1977.

9. Klotz, U., Avant, G.R., Hoyumpa, A., Schenker, S., and Wilkinson, G.R. The effects of age and liver disease on the disposition and elimination of diazepam in adult man. *J. of Clin. Investigation* 55:347, 1975.

10. Miller, A.K., Adir, J., and Vestal, R.E. Tolbutamide binding to plasma proteins of young and old human subjects. *J. Pharm. Sci.* 67:1192, 1978.

11. Hayes, M.J., Langman, M.J.S., and Short, A.H. Changes in drug metabolism with increasing age. 2. Phenytoin clearance and protein binding. *Br. J. Clin. Pharmacol.* 2:73, 1975.

12. O'Malley, K., Crooks, J., Duke, E., and Stevenson, I.H. Effect of age and sex on human drug metabolism. *Br. Med. J.* 3:607, 1971.

13. Swift, C.G., Homeida, M., Halliwell, M., and Roberts, C.J.C. Antipyrine disposition and liver size in the elderly. *Eur. J. Clin. Pharmacol.* 14:149, 1978.

14. Wood, A.J.J., Vestal, R.E., Wilkinson, G.R., Branch, R.A., and Shand, D.G. The effects of aging and cigarette smoking on the elimination of antipyrine and indocyanine gree. *Clin. Pharmacol. Ther.* 26:16, 1979.

15. Jusko, W.J., Koup, J.R., Vance, J.W., Schentag, J.J., and Kuritzky, P. Intravenous theophylline: Nomogram guidelines. *Ann. Intern. Med.* 86:400, 1977.

16. Bellville, J.W., Forrest, W.H., Miller, E., and Brown, B.W. Influence of age on pain relief from analgesics. A study of postoperative patients. *JAMA* 217:1835, 1971.

17. Greenblatt, D.J., Allen, M.D., and Shader, R.I. Toxicity of high-dose flurazepam in the elderly. *Clin. Pharmacol. and Ther.* 21:355, 1977.

18. Castleden, C.M., George, C.E., Marcer, D., and Hallett, C. Increased sensitivity to nitrazepam in old age. *Br. Med. J.* 1:10, 1977.

19. Reidenberg, M.M., Levy, M., Warner, H., Coutinho, C.B., Schwartz, M.A., Yu, G., and Cheriplco, J. The relationship between diazepam dose, plasma

level, age and central nervous system depression in adults. *Clin. Pharmacol. Ther.* 23:371, 1978.

20. Vestal, R.E., Wood, A.J.J., and Shand, D.G. Reduced β-adrenoceptor sensitivity in the elderly. *Clin. Pharmacol. Ther.* 26:181, 1979.

21. Schocken, D. and Roth, G. Reduced beta-adrenergic receptor concentrations in aging man. *Nature* 267:856, 1977.

25

Alterations that Occur in the Hearts of Healthy Men and Animals in Senescence

Edward G. Lakatta, M.D.

"Like presbyopia, presbycardia (myocardial senescence) is a functional change associated with minimal anatomic alteration, which may begin soon after maturity and may lead to loss of adaptation of the aging tissue to its more exacting burdens" [1]. In the 35 years since Dock postulated that the senescent heart was deficient in adaptive capacity, several studies have delineated anatomical and functional changes that occur in the heart as a result of advancing age. In some instances, these studies have also elucidated mechanisms that may underlie these age-related changes [2-5]. The extent to which the results of such investigations reflect the "normal" aging process is determined by the level of certainty regarding the absence of specific disease, that is, occult coronary disease. In studies of normal aged human beings, it is of particular importance to detect the presence of coronary disease, which exists in 50% to 70% of persons aged 60 and 80 [6]. In order to accomplish this, it is often necessary to employ stress to the cardiovascular system. Additional selective criteria, for example, the limit of blood pressure regarded as normal at a given age, physical fitness, nutrition, and life style, should also be considered in the interpretation of the results of investigations of "normal" aging of the cardiovascular system.

Within the past decade, the advent of ultrasound as a clinical research tool has enabled noninvasive study of some functional and morphologic aspects of the heart in men of all ages [7]. Studies utilizing this technique have been performed on participants of the Baltimore Longitudinal Study, a well-characterized population ranging from ages 25 to 85 [8]. Subjects who had a history of cardiac disease or who exhibited signs of cardiac disease by physical examination, chest x-ray, and resting electrocardiography were excluded from the analysis. In addition, those subjects whose electrocardiogram during maximal treadmill exercise exhibited positive or borderline positive changes, indicative of latent coronary artery disease, were also excluded. Subjects who had systolic blood pressures greater than 150 mm Hg and diastolic pressures greater than 90 mm Hg were likewise excluded from this study. However, it is important to note that even in this select group, both systolic and mean blood pressure significantly increased from ages 20 to 80. The results of this study indicated that while left ventricular dimensions are unaltered with aging, left ventricular wall thickness, both end diastolic and end systolic, increases as a function of age.

In men aged 65 to 80, wall thickness was 30% greater than in the younger age groups. This moderate increase in left ventricular thickness with increasing age in normal human beings has also been demonstrated in two additional studies utilizing this technique [9,10]. These findings are in contrast to the notion that the heart atrophies in normal human beings with advancing age [1]. At rest, stroke output and total cardiac output decline or are unaltered with advancing age [2]. However, these parameters fail to account for internal work and impedance to ejection, which are major components of total cardiac work. It has long been recognized that both systolic and mean blood pressure increase with age, both at rest and during exercise, and constitute an age-related load on the heart. The structure, size, and reactivity of the arterial bed can affect myocardial performance by increasing the impedance to left ventricular ejection. The latter is a function of central aortic compliance or stiffness, the systemic vascular resistance, the reflected pressure waves, and the inertial properties of the blood. Age changes have been identified in the first two factors.

For at least a century, it has been recognized that arterial walls stiffen with age in both animals and human beings. Aortas as well as small arteries exhibit a greater resistance to deformation with age. It should be emphasized that the age change in vascular stiffness is attributed to a diffuse process that occurs in the vessel wall and that cannot be explained on the basis of atherosclerosis [2]. When vascular impedance is high, a higher systolic pressure must be developed and more work done by the left ventricle. Systolic left ventricular wall tension and myocardial oxygen consumption increase substantially as a result of the increase in systolic pressure. As a result of the increase in vascular input impedance, the heart of the older individual can be less able to augment cardiac output. In circumstances when stroke volume falls, as during many arrhythmias, organ perfusion can also be compromised to a greater extent in the aged than in younger adults, as a result of vessels that are stiffer and less capable of vasoregulation.

It is of interest to determine whether the age-related increase in left ventricular wall thickness is accompanied by alterations in function. At rest, the fractional shortening of the minor semiaxis, a correlate of ejection fraction and thus a measure of pump function, is not age related in this population. The velocity of circumferential shortening, an ejection phase index of myocardial performance, is also not a function of age in individuals in the resting state [8]. The early diastolic filling rate, however, as reflected in the E-F slope of the mitral valve, progressively decreases with age. A similar decrease in filling rate is also present in hypertrophied hearts in many disease states. Possible mechanisms for a diminished filling rate in the aged heart include age-related alterations in the mitral valve, increased myocardial stiffness [2], and prolonged duration of contraction, which has been demonstrated in both intact hearts and cardiac muscle of senescent animals [3].

According to our current understanding of the contraction-relaxation cycle, for an activated cardiac muscle to relax, the intracellular concentration of free Ca^{++}, the activator substance, must be reduced to below threshold levels. In mammalian cardiac muscle, this is accomplished in large degree by sequestration of Ca^{++} by the sarcoplasmic reticulum. Studies have indicated that these membranes isolated from hearts of senescent rats sequester Ca^{++} at a reduced rate compared to those from hearts of adult animals [11]. This observation provides a plausible explanation on a cellular level for prolonged activation in cardiac muscle in animals and prolonged isometric relaxation in humans.

While the diminished filling rate of the senescent heart may not be important in cardiac performance at rest, when the diastolic filling time is shortened, such as during tachycardia, reduced filling could compromise stroke output and lead to a lower threshold for dyspnea in elderly man compared to his younger adult counterpart. Additional studies during stress, however, are required to test this hypothesis.

It has been well documented that maximum cardiac output and oxygen consumption in humans diminish with advancing age [2]. It is not clear, however, to what extent the age deficit in cardiovascular performance is attributed to an age difference in loading of the heart during exercise [4]. Ultrasound studies indicate that the heart in normal elderly persons reacts like the heart of young individuals in response to an increase in afterload of a 20 mm Hg increase in mean blood pressure induced by phenylephrine [12]. However, in the presence of β-adrenergic blockade, ventricular dilation occurred in response to the increased afterload in the elderly but not in the younger adults, suggesting an intrinsic weakness of cardiac muscle in the senescent heart.

During semisupine exercise that resulted in a heart rate of 100 beats/min, VCF (velocity of circumferential fiber shortening) measured echocardiographically increased in younger men but failed to increase in elderly men [13]. Since in this protocol, end diastolic heart dimension did not change and blood pressure changed equally in both age groups, the results appear to indicate a diminished reserve or intrinsic weakness in the heart of normal elderly men. One possible mechanism for the diminished reserve is a diminished response of cardiac muscle to catecholamines secreted during exercise. Such a diminution has been demonstrated in isolated rat cardiac muscle [14,15]. In addition, a series of studies in intact animals and humans measuring a variety of hemodynamic responses suggest that the cardiovascular response to catecholamines declines in senesence [4]. Much additional study is required, however, in order to elucidate mechanisms for these age-related differences.

In summary, it seems fair to conclude that at rest the moderate cardiac hypertrophy that occurs with advancing age, while accompanied by reduced filling in early diastole, does not impair cardiac function. Thus, as such, no such entity as *symptomatic* senile cardiomyopathy exists. In response to hemodynamic stress, however, age-related changes in the cardiovascular system, both structural and functional, have an impact on cardiovascular performance. It would seem likely that these age-related changes in the heart also modify the accommodation of the cardiovascular system to specific pathologic cardiovascular disease states, and thus have an impact on the clinical presentation of specific cardiovascular disease entities in the elderly. In this context, presbycardia [1] appears to be a reality.

References

1. Dock, W. Presbycardia, or aging of the myocardium. *N.Y. State J. Med.* 45:983, 1945.
2. Gerstenblith, G., Lakatta, E.G., and Weisfeldt, M.L. Age changes in myocardial function and exercise response. *Prog. Cardiovascular Dis.* 19:1, 1976.
3. Lakatta, E.G., Alterations in the cardiovascular system that occur in advanced age. *Federation Proc.* 38:163, 1970.
4. Lakatta, E.G. Age-related alterations in the cardiovascular response to adrenergic mediated stress. *Federation Proc.* (in press).
5. Weisfeldt, M.L. (Ed.). *The Heart in Old Age: Its Function and Response to Stress.* New York: Raven Press, 1980.
6. Lakatta, E.G. and Gerstenblith, G. Cardiovascular gerontology. In J.W. Rowe (Ed.) *Textbook on Geriatric Medicine.* Boston: Little Brown and Co., (in press).
7. Feigenbaum, H. *Echocardiography* (2nd Ed.) Philadelphia: Lea & Febiger, 1976.
8. Gerstenblith, G., Frederiksen, J., Yin, F.C.P., Fortuin, E.G., Lakatta, E.G., and Weisfeldt, M.L. Echocardiographic assessment of a normal adult aging population. *Circulation* 56:273, 1977.
9. Sjogren, A.L. Left ventricular wall thickness determined by ultrasound in 100 subjects without heart disease. *Chest* 60:341, 1971.
10. Savage, D.D., Drayer, J.I.M., Henry, W.L., Mathews, Jr., E.C., Ware, J.H., Gardin, J.M., Cohen, E.R., Epstein, S.R., and Laragh, J.H. Echocardiographic assessment of cardiac anatomy and function in hypertensive subjects. *Circulation* 59:623, 1979.
11. Froehlich, J.P., Lakatta, E.G., Bear, E., Spurgeon, H.A., Weisfeldt, M.L., and Gerstenblith, G., Studies of sarcoplasmic reticulum function and contraction duration in young and aged rat myocardium. *J. Mol. Cell. Cardio.* 10:427, 1978.
12. Sugishita, Y., and Koseki, S. Dynamic exercise echocardiography. *Circulation* 60:743, 1979.
14. Lakatta, E.G., Gerstenblith, G., Angell, C.S., Shock, N.W., and Weisfeldt, M.L. Diminished inotropic response of aged myocardium to catecholamines. *Circulation Res.* 36:262, 1975.

15. Guarnieri, T., Filburn, C., Zitnik, G., Roth, G., and Lakatta, E.G., contractile and biochemical correlates of beta-adreneric stimulation of the aged heart. *Amer. J. Physiol.* 239:H501, 1980.

26 The Human Brain in Normal Aging and in Dementia

Dennis J. Selkoe, M.D.

Although the events underlying age-related neuronal attrition remain poorly understood, important progress in our clinical and neurobiological understanding of the pathogenesis of senile dementia has occurred in the past two decades. This fact and the likelihood of accelerated progress in the coming decade are indeed welcome developments. The maturing of our population and the decline in mortality from the major fatal diseases of late life, for example, cerebrovascular disorders [1], compel us to seek solutions to the emerging public health problem of senile dementia [2,3]. We will review the changing notions of senile dementia and its relationship to normal aging and then focus on recent research developments and their implications for future therapies.

Current Understanding of Senile Dementia

Perhaps the most important alteration in our thinking about late-life dementia is the conclusion that atherosclerotic disease of the cerebral vasculature is not the major cause of progressive impairment of memory and other intellectual functions during aging. This conclusion results from extensive neuropathological studies carried out in several laboratories on both sides of the Atlantic. These have shown that the correlation between cerebral atherosclerosis and the presence and degree of senile dementia is not strong. However, a significant minority of the demented elderly have one or more macroscopically visible areas of hemispheral infarction. In carefully documented clinicopathological series [4,5], approximately 10% to 20% of demented patients over age 65 showed ischemic infarction in the absence of neurofibrillary changes as the major neuropathological finding. While the majority of patients with senile dementia show little or no tissue destroyed by ischemia, elderly subjects with extensive (> 100 cc) cerebral infarction are almost invariably demented to some degree.

It has become clear that patients with what is now referred to as multi-infarct dementia can be separated from the majority with degenerative dementia on the basis of the step-wise clinical evolution of the intellectual deficits, the positive physical findings, and cerebral blood flow studies. Hachinski and co-workers [6] have divided their patients with senile dementia into two groups on the basis of a previously validated "ischemic score": primary degenerative dementia (Alzheimer disease, AD) with no clinical evidence of vascular symptoms

149

or signs and multi-infarct dementia (MID) with high ischemic scores. The degree
of dementia, assessed by both a dementia scale based on clinical symptoms and
by a cognitive test, was the same in the two groups. Measurement of total and
regional cerebral blood flow (CBF) using the Xenon-133 method revealed significant decreases in total hemispheral flow, initial flow and fast flow (flow
through fast-clearing tissue, primarily gray matter) in the MID group only. There
were no significant changes in these parameters in the AD patients. However, the
portion of brain tissue showing fast flow (an approximation of gray matter volume) was significantly reduced from 49% in controls to approximately 42% in
both MID and AD patients. Among MID patients, there was a significant inverse
correlation between mean fast flow and test scores, whereas no such relationship
was evident in the degenerative group. The reactivity of cerebral vessels to hypo-
capnia was normal in both groups. One can conclude that there is a close relationship between the degree of dementia and the decrease in gray matter blood
flow when cerebrovascular disease rather than neuronal degeneration is the
apparent cause of the dementia. Since CBF is measured per 100 g of brain tissue,
loss of cortical neurons in AD patients would not of itself decrease flow as long
as the metabolic demands of the remaining brain were near normal.

Another important reinterpretation in our practical understanding of the
dementias is the evidence, now widely accepted, that presenile dementia of the
AD type and degenerative senile dementia are indistinguishable on clinical,
neuropathologic, or ultrastructural grounds. The major pathologic findings of
cortical atrophy with marked neuronal loss, intraneuronal neurofibrillary tangles, extraneuronal neuritic (or senile) plaques, and granulovacuolar degeneration
have long been recognized as identical in patients with clinical onset before
age 65 (presenile) or after age 65 (senile). Although most investigators in the
field now use the term Alzheimer disease for both forms, the Commission on
Nosology of the recent NIH workshop conference on Alzheimer disease recommended use of the term *Alzheimer disease* in the presenium and the term *senile
dementia of the Alzheimer type* in the senium, to avoid prejudging the etiologic
identity of these forms [7].

It appears that biochemical alterations in AD brain tissue, such as the recently described deficiency of cholinergic enzymes (see below), are present both
in presenile and senile cases. The epidemiologic question of whether the incidence of the disorder rises gradually with age, suggesting a single pathogenetic
process, or has a bimodal age distribution before and after age 65 has not yet
been settled.

A recurring and as yet unsettled issue in the study of human neuronal
aging has been the relationship of the degenerative dementias to normal senescence. Many workers consider senile dementia a disease process that can be
separated from the age-related psychometric and neuropathologic changes occurring in a large percentage of the elderly. The notion that senile dementia is an
accelerated form of "benign senescent forgetfulness" and that most aged indi-

viduals would develop Alzheimer disease if they lived long enough is not borne out by available data [8]. Two follow-up studies of a total of 800 institutionalized patients with average ages at initial evaluation of 75 and 80 years, respectively, revealed that only a small percentage of patients originally free of senile dementia developed the disease during the following 10 years [9,10]. This preservation of functional integrity in a large majority of the elderly has been supported by other studies. The periodic inability of many elderly individuals to recall certain unimportant data about an event, while readily recalling the event itself, suggests a variable impairment of recall that is qualitatively distinct from the total erasure of large portions of memory seen in the demented patient. Another important difference is that the "benign" type of memory change is not correlated with the shortened survival time characteristic of Alzheimer disease [8]. The important clinical observation that the incidence of senile dementia is considerably higher in women than would be expected from their greater longevity further serves to separate AD patients from the general aged population.

In addition to such clinical evidence, neuropathologic and biochemical studies point to clear distinctions between the estimated 5% to 12% of individuals over age 65 who are demented [11] and the elderly population at large.

Changes in the Brain with Aging and Dementia

Several morphological changes have long been known to occur in the cerebral cortex of both aged and demented individuals. The most obvious gross alteration is a 10% to 12% decline in total brain weight during normal senescence compared to the mature adult, associated primarily with thinning of the cerebral cortex and compensatory dilation of the lateral ventricles. Although severely demented patients often have greater loss of cortical tissue than age-matched nondemented individuals, this is not always the case. In this regard, several recent studies have pointed out the inadequacy of present computed tomographic (CT) scanning methods in clearly distinguishing normal gyral atrophy from that occurring in dementia. It is believed that cortical thinning is largely the result of progressive neuronal loss. Several groups, using semiquantitative techniques, have demonstrated a steady attrition of nerve cells that occurs in the normal adult population throughout life, both in lower mammals and in humans. Brody [12] found an approximately 50% loss of cortical neurons between the ages of 20 and 90. In Alzheimer disease, although neuronal loss is classically described, recent automated cell counts employing an image analyzing computer seem to show as wide a scatter in neuronal counts per unit cortex from senile Alzheimer disease patients as from aged controls, with few or no cases of senile dementia thus far reported showing cell counts below the nondemented population [4]. Preliminary results from other laboratories using automated counting appear to confirm the fact that at least mean neuronal loss per unit area of frontal and temporal cortex is similar in senile dementia and normal aging. However, no such study has corrected counts for total volume of cortex in each brain. Since available information points strongly to a decrease in cortical volume with age, normal cell loss can be even more marked than these counts have shown. Furthermore, greater atrophy in Alzheimer disease than in normal aged cortex might lead to a smaller total neuronal population in the former condition. Such a difference in mean cortical atrophy, however, has not yet been quantitatively demonstrated.

As is well known, the most prevalent microscopic alterations of human brain found in Alzheimer disease and in normal individuals of great age are the neuritic, or senile, plaque and the neurofibrillary tangle. The neuritic plaque is a cortical lesion consisting of many abnormal neuritic processes lying in an extracellular matrix that is largely composed of amyloid. The enlarged processes in this structure have been shown to be both presynaptic and postsynaptic elements, but especially, axonal boutons that contain fibrous organelles identical to those of the neurofibrillary tangle, as well as degenerating lysosomes and mitochondria. The neurofibrillary tangle, on the other hand, is a wholly intracellular lesion that consists of a tangled mass of abnormal cytoplasmic fibrils that are highly argyrophilic when stained with silver preparations, and then resemble a steel wool pad. The ultrastructure of the abnormal fibers found in these two classical lesions of Alzheimer disease has been the subject of some debate. There is now growing agreement that the abnormal organelles are made up of a pair of helically wound 9 nm to 10 nm filaments, rather than a pinched or "twisted" microtubule-like structure, as was previously believed. This morphological issue has considerable importance for the interpretation of protein chemical studies, which our laboratory and others have been carrying out on Alzheimer tissue.

The third classical lesion of Alzheimer disease, granulovacuolar degeneration of cortical neurons, is inconsistently seen in such brains and found less frequently in the normal aged brain. The granulovacuolar change does not involve abnormalities of fibrous proteins.

Although neurofibrillary degeneration of the perikarya and the neuropil is most marked and specific in Alzheimer disease, it is also found in several other neurological disorders that have dementia as a prominent feature. These include postencephalitic Parkinson disease, the parkinsonism-dementia complex found in remarkably high incidence in the Chamorro Indians on Guam, and, occasionally, the slow measles virus infection, subacute sclerosing panencephalitis. Of particular interest is the development of a neurofibrillary degeneration that is ultrastructurally identical to Alzheimer disease in a high proportion of patients with Down syndrome (trisomy 21) after the third decade. It is noteworthy that the unusual paired helical filaments of the Alzheimer neurofibrillary tangle and the neuritic plaque occur only in the human and only in brain. Lesions that resemble primitive senile plaques have been reported in the cortex of very old monkeys and dogs. However, the fine structure of such plaques is clearly distinguishable from the human change by the absence of the twisted fibrous organelles.

One may question the importance of neurofibrillary change in the pathogenesis of memory loss and dementia when these lesions are also the most important microscopic changes found in the brains of intellectually normal old people. However, recent quantitative histopathological studies [4,13,14] have demonstrated very significant differences in the density and distribution of plaques and tangle in cortex between the normal aged and those with the clinical syndrome of Alzheimer disease. The quantitative analyses of Tomlinson and others have documented the steady accumulation of neuritic plaques and neurofibrillary tangles with advancing age. Microscopic sections of cortex reveal small numbers of neuritic plaques in approximately 15% of normals by age 50, in roughly 50% by age 70, and in 75% by age 90 [14]. Although the percentages may seem impressive, the actual number of plaques per microscopic field in individuals who have been carefully tested and found to have normal intellect within 6 months of death is very low, less than 5 plaques per field in 70% of such subjects and less than 10 plaques per field in 90%. The mean plaque count in nondemented subjects over age 65 is only 3 per field, compared to 15 per field in demented patients of similar age (difference significant at $p < 0.001$) [4]. Moreover, within the nondemented group, those patients who made minimal errors on intellectual testing had mean plaque counts of 5.6 per field compared to only 1.5 in those with full preservation of mental status. The authors of these studies have further pointed out that in mentally normal subjects showing plaque formation, the lesions are discrete and widely separated, with only middle cortical layers involved, whereas in the demented, plaques tend to cluster and overlap, with involvement of all layers and the appearance of abnormal neuropil between plaques.

A similar situation obtains for the neurofibrillary tangle (NFT). These intraneuronal lesions can be found in small numbers in the brains of a few normals in middle age and in a majority after the age of 65. By age 90, few patients are devoid of NFTs. However, the lesions in controls are few in number and largely confined to hippocampus and amygdala. Even there, scanning light microscopy has documented that the number of tangle-bearing hippocampal neurons is 6 to 40 times greater in Alzheimer disease than in age-matched controls [13]. Ball has observed that the maximum density of neurofibrillary tangles and granulovacuolar degeneration in Alzheimer hippocampus occurred in areas that had already sustained the greatest cell loss, thus augmenting the significance of these lesions in the small number of surviving neurons]14]. A pattern of moderate or large numbers of tangles widely scattered throughout neocortex is totally restricted to demented patients.

One may conclude that the distinctions between neuronal lesions in Alzheimer dementia and in the nondemented elderly are quantitative and topographic rather than qualitative. The endogenous and/or exogenous factors that lead to widespread and progressive fibrillary degeneration of neuronal perikarya and their processes in certain individuals are not yet understood. It is apparent, however, that neurofibrillary change is pathogenetically associated with, or is a clear marker for, a gross abnormality of neuronal function which is clinically expressed as disordered memory and intellect.

Recent Research Developments
in the Study of Senile Dementia

Investigation of presenile and senile dementia of the Alzheimer type continues to involve the pursuit of widely divergent leads, as is appropriate for a disease without even a tentative hypothesis as to etiology. In the space available here, we will be able to review only selected, recent studies. We are, therefore, forced to exclude some areas of research that may turn out to have considerable relevance in ultimately deciphering the mechanisms of age-related neuronal attrition.

Biochemical Studies

Among various biochemical investigations of Alzheimer brain tissue in recent years, two areas of study have aroused particular interest: the analysis of neuro-transmitter alterations and the macromolecular chemistry of the abnormal neuronal filaments found in degenerating neurons. The study of changes in synaptic transmitters took on new interest in 1976 with the finding by three independent groups in Great Britain of a marked and selective abnormality of the presynaptic cholinergic system in cortex affected with Alzheimer disease [17-19]. Levels of choline acetyl transferase (CAT), the principal synthetic enzyme for acetylcholine, are reduced by 50% to 90% in hippocampus, amygdala, and neocortex, with lesser reductions in deep gray nuclei. Although initial determinations were made in autopsied cortex, agonal or postmortem autolysis was eliminated by the finding of normal activity of glutamic acid decarboxylase (GAD), an enzyme particularly sensitive to antemortem hypoxia [17]. Subsequently, biopsied cortex in Alzheimer disease showed a similar marked decrease in CAT activity with preservation of GAD [19]. Levels of acetylcholinesterase (AChE) are also dramatically reduced in limbic and neocortex. Regions of cerebral cortex showing the greatest reductions in CAT and AChE activity correlate roughly with areas of maximum neurofibrillary pathology [17]. Recently, Perry and coworkers [20] have reported that the decline of CAT can be quantitatively correlated with the density of neuritic plaques in cortex. Preliminary studies show no significant decrease in activity of the catecholamine transmitter enzymes, tyrosine hydroxylase, aromatic amino acid decarboxylase, dopamine-p-hydroxylase and monoamine exidase, thus emphasizing the apparent selective vulnerability of cholinergic neurons in this disease.

Since CAT is a marker for presynaptic cholinergic nerve endings, these biochemical results appear to correlate with the abnormalities of presynaptic axon terminals in cortex affected with Alzheimer disease. On the postsynaptic side, in contrast, muscarinic cholinergic receptor binding activity is the same as in age-matched controls [16]. Two hypotheses can be raised: (1) the reductions in CAT and AChE activities can represent degeneration of cholinergic nerve terminals rather than parent cell bodies, thus explaining the apparent lack of specific perikaryal loss found by automated counting; and (2) the use of central anticholinesterases or, preferably, cholinergic agonists offers a rational hope for therapeutic benefit.

The initial attempts at therapy using cholinergic agents that these studies spawned have increased in the past two years, thus far without convincing positive results. Orally administered choline salts have been shown to significantly increase plasma and cerebrospinal fluid choline levels in humans but appear to cause little or no improvement in memory or most cognitive functions in patients with moderate or advanced Alzheimer disease. Likewise, deanol, an agent that increases brain acetylcholine levels, and physostigmine, the centrally acting anticholinesterase, have generally failed to improve memory in Alzheimer patients. We may, however, be in the situation faced by investigators studying dopaminergic treatment in Parkinson disease prior to the use of high-dose prolonged L-dopa therapy. Several sustained trials of cholinergic agents in patients with early dementia are currently underway.

The macromolecular events that lead to selective abiotrophy of neurons in aging and dementia, and therefore presumably precede neurotransmitter deficiencies, are almost entirely unknown. Biochemical investigation into the nature of the plaques and tangles that are the hallmarks of Alzheimer disease is in its formative stages. A major obstacle to identification of the fibrous protein that forms the abnormal paired helical filaments found in both of these lesions has been the difficulty in characterizing completely the normal 10 nm neuronal filaments. Iqbal and colleagues [19] have identified a 50,000 MW protein as the presumptive subunit of the paired helical filaments (PHF). The interpretation of their finding is complicated by the fact that this is also the molecular weight of the subunit of the 10 nm glial filament characteristic of astroglia. Since the fractions enriched in neurofibrillary tangles, and thus PHF, may include some glial material from the gliotic cortical areas containing the tangles, the proposed PHF subunit could represent a protein of glial rather than neuronal origin. In our laboratory, we have not yet confirmed an augmentation of the 50,000 MW protein in isolated neuronal fractions from Alzheimer brain enriched in neurofibrillary tangles. Some neuronal fractions from affected Alzheimer cortex have been shown by us to contain a marked augmentation of a 20,000 MW protein compared to fractions from age-matched normal and Huntington disease brains [20]. The identity of this new protein alteration is not yet clear, but initial evidence suggests it is not directly related to the paired helical filaments themselves. Work is presently underway to try to characterize further the protein composition of degenerating, PHF-bearing neurons in Alzheimer disease by bio-chemical and immunological means.

An allied approach to the problem of fibrillary degeneration of neurons has involved studies of experimental models in which various neurotoxins can in-duce large masses of structurally normal-appearing 10 nm neurofilaments in mammalian neurons. An animal model that has aroused particular interest is the intracerebral or cisternal injection of aluminum ions, which produce striking intra-neuronal bundles of neurofilaments accompanied by a progressive fatal encepha-lomyelopathy. It should be noted that the aluminum-induced filaments are not helically wound in the fashion of the PHF of Alzheimer disease. Crapper and colleagues [21] studied the early course of the intoxication, when the animals were asymptomatic, and found that their performance on a task requiring retention of new information (short-term memory) progressively declined and that the level of performance correlated with cortical aluminum levels. Neurons undergoing such neurofibrillary degeneration induced by aluminum have now been isolated and their filaments have been shown by biochemical and immuno-logic techniques to be highly similar if not identical to normally occurring 10 nm neuronal filaments [22]. What has made this model appear more intrigu-ing has been the finding by Crapper et al. [21] of a several-fold elevation of human cortical aluminum levels in topographical relationship to the neurofibril-lary tangles in Alzheimer disease. The source of the aluminum and its potential etiologic relevance, if any, to the dementia remain obscure. A serious question remains as to whether aluminum ions, if they are confirmed as excessive in Alzheimer cortex, merely accumulate there as a secondary phenomenon, perhaps following some earlier pathologic change of neuronal membranes.

Neuropathologic Studies

In addition to the various light-microscopic and ultrastructual observations on Alzheimer brain tissue reviewed earlier, mention should be made of recent studies indicating marked alterations of neuronal processes in Alzheimer disease. Changes in neuronal processes, as opposed to lesions of the cell bodies, have evoked increasing interest as a possible morphologic correlate of documented changes in synaptic biochemistry. A decrease in the extent of cortical dendritic arborization and in the density of dendritic spines as a function of age was re-ported by Scheibel and coworkers in neocortex and limbic cortex of normal humans [23]. Similar studies in lower mammals by these authors have shown few alterations in neocortex but widespread and progressive age-related dendritic changes in many brainstem and spinal-cord neurons [24]. Recently, however, Buell and Coleman [25] have reported computer-microscope analyses of autop-sied parahippocampal cortex that do not document loss of dendritic extent in normal human cortex with aging, but rather the opposite. These authors reported an unexpected growth of the terminal dendritic tree in normal human cortex between the ages of 50 and 80. Their results provide evidence of plasticity in the mature and aged human brain. In contrast, they found evidence of shrinkage of dendritic arbor (fewer and shorter terminal dendritic segments) in patients with documented senile dementia. The latter finding is in general agreement with earlier morphometric studies of human hippocampus and frontal cortex in presenile and senile dementia suggesting a 25% to 50% loss of dendritic spines compared to age-matched controls [26]. Buell and Coleman postulate that the aging brain can contain one population of neurons that dies and regresses and another that survives and grows. They suggest that the latter appears to be the dominant population in aging without dementia. Further work in this important area will be needed to clarify the difference in findings of the various investigators.

Virologic Studies

The possibility of viral etiologies for various neuronal abiotrophies of late life has become increasingly attractive in the decade since the discovery that Creutzfeldt-Jakob disease is caused by a transmissible, filterable agent. Neither the identity of this virus nor the natural mode of transmission have been established. In the case of Alzheimer disease, there is at present only limited and circumstantial evidence to support a viral etiology. Viral-like particles have not been found in brain affected with Alzheimer disease, although this appears to be characteristic for slow infections caused by unconventional viruses (for example, Kuru and Creutzfeldt-Jakob disease) [27]. The clinical syndrome and neuropathology of Alzheimer disease are generally distinguishable from the known slow-virus encephalopathies of humans. However, neurofibrillary tangles that are ultrastructurally identical to those in Alzheimer disease have been found in postencephalitic parkinsonism and in rare, long-surviving cases of subacute sclerosing panencephalitis. In two cases of familial Alzheimer disease, brain injected into New World monkeys produced, after a two-year latent period, a clinical and pathologic syndrome typical of the primate subacute spongiform encephalopathy that occurs after inoculation of Creutzfeld-Jakob tissue [27]. However, no histologic features of Alzheimer disease were produced. Brain tissue from more than forty classical sporadic cases of Alzheimer disease has now been inoculated into a variety of primates, and, to date, no animal has developed any neurologic disease, despite latent intervals of up to seven years in some instances (C.J. Gibbs, Jr., personal communication).

Perhaps the strongest link to a viral process comes from the recent report of DeBoni and Crapper that small numbers of paired helical filaments can be found in the processes of cultured human fetal cortical neurons exposed to saline extracts of a brain with Alzheimer disease [28]. Although several important control experiments have yet to be reported, this finding raises the possibility of a transmissible agent or toxin as a cause of human neurofibrillary degeneration. An additional laboratory model of potential relevance is the scrapie-exposed mouse. Certain susceptible strains of inbred female mice have been shown to develop argyrophilic neuritic plaques in gray matter almost two years after brain inoculation with the agent causing scrapie, a naturally occurring slow-virus infection of sheep [29]. Electron microscopy of these induced lesions shows them to be highly similar to classical senile plaques of humans, although their abnormal neurites do not contain the paired helical filaments seen in Alzheimer disease.

Conclusion

The application of newer techniques in neuronal cell biology and biochemistry has provided some intriguing clues to the pathogenesis of Alzheimer disease. Yet clear understanding of the etiology of this common and devastating disorder is not at hand. That this should be so is not surprising, since clinical and laboratory investigations of the late-life dementias are in their infancy compared to the cumulative research efforts that have been directed at still-unresolved neurologic disorders, such as multiple sclerosis. It is tantalizing to speculate that endogenous (genetic) or exogenous (toxic) factors may act (singly or together) on the nerve cell's nuclear apparatus, thereby causing accumulation of altered proteins, expressed morphologically as paired helical filaments, which in turn may interfere with neuronal metabolism and transport (or vice versa), thus affecting maintenance of the cell's axons and dendrites and leading ultimately to a deficiency of presynaptic transmitters, cholinergic or otherwise. Since such a relationship remains entirely unproven, one must be satisfied with the inevitable multifactorial hypothesis of the pathogenesis of Alzheimer disease at present.

Fortunately, the lack of an etiologic understanding does not preclude advances in the therapy of the disorder. The very recent progress in synaptic biochemistry has led to the current formative trials of agents such as lecithin and physostigmine. One can only hope that additional agents capable of affecting synaptic and other altered functions in Alzheimer tissue will become available as the enormous problem of senile dementia achieves increasing recognition in the biomedical and lay communities.

References

1. Garraway, W.M., Whisnont, J.P., Fulan, A.J., et al. The declining incidence of stroke. *N. Eng. J. Med.* 300:449, 1979.

2. Plum, F. Dementia: an approaching epidemic. *Nature* 279:372, 1979.

3. Katzman, R. The prevalence and malignancy of Alzheimer disease. *Arch. Neurol.* 33:217, 1976.

4. Tomlinson, B.F. and Henderson, G. Some quantitative cerebral findings in normal and demented old people. In R.D. Terry and S. Gershon (Eds.) *Neurobiology of Aging,* New York: Raven Press, 1976.

5. Corsellis, J. *Mental Illness and the Aging Brain.* London: Oxford University Press, 1962.

6. Hachinski, V.C., Hiff, L.D., Zillika, E., et al. Cerebral blood flow in dementia. *Arch. Neurol.* 32:632, 1975.

7. Katzman, R., Terry, R.D., and Beck, K.L. (Eds.) *Alzheimer's Disease: Senile Dementia and Related Disorders.* New York: Raven Press, 1978.

8. Kral, V.A. Senescent forgetfulness: benign and malignant. *Can. Med. Assoc. J.* 86:257, 1962.

9. Kral, V.A. Memory disorders in old age and senility. In G.A. Talland and N.C. Waugh (Eds.), *The Pathology of Memory.* New York: Academic Press, 1969.

10. Kral, V.A. and Muellen, H. Memory dysfunction: a prognostic indicator in geriatric patients. *Can. Psych. Assoc. J.* 11:343, 1966.

11. Terry, R.D. Dementia: a brief and selective review. *Arch. Neurol.* 33:1, 1976.

12. Brody, H. Organization of the cerebral cortex. III. A study of aging in cerebral cortex. *J. Comp. Neurol.* 102:511, 1955.

13. Ball, M.J. Neurofibrillary tangles and the pathogenesis of dementia: A quantitative time study. *Neuropath. Appl. Neurobiol.* 2:294, 1976.

14. Ball, M.J. Neuronal loss, neurofibrillary tangles and granulovacuolar degeneration in the hippocampus with aging and dementia. A quantitative study. *Acta Neuropath.* 37:111, 1977.

15. Davis, P. and Maloney, A.J.F. Selective loss of central cholinergic neurons in Alzheimer's disease. *Lancet* 2:1403, 1976.

16. Perry, E.K., Perry, R.H., Blessed, G., et al. Necropsy evidence of central nervous system cholinergic deficits in senile dementia. *Lancet* 1:189, 1977.

17. Spillane, J.A., White, P., Goodhardt, M.J., et al. Selective vulnerability of neurons in organic dementia. *Nature* 266:558, 1977.

18. Perry, E.K., Tomlinson, B.E., Blessed, G., et al. Correlation of cholinergic abnormalities with senile plaques and mental test scores in senile dementia. *Brit. Med. J.* 2:1457, 1978.

19. Iqbal, L., Wisniewski, H.M., Shelanski, M.L., et al. Protein changes in senile dementia. *Brain Res.* 77:337, 1974.

20. Selkow, D.J. Altered protein composition of isolated human cortical neurons in Alzheimer's disease. *Annals Neurol.* 8:468, 1980.

21. Crapper, D.R., Krishman, S.S., and Dalton, A.J. Brain aluminum distribution in Alzheimer's disease and experimental neurofibrillary degeneration. *Science* 180:511, 1973.

22. Selkoe, D.J., Liem, R.K.H., Yen, S.H., and Shelanski, M.L. Biochemical and immunological characterization of neurofilaments in experimental neurofibrillary degeneration induced by aluminum. *Brain Res.* 163:235, 1979.

23. Scheibel, M.T., Lindsay, R.D., Tomiyasu, U., et al. Progressive dendritic changes in the aging human limbic system. *Exp. Neurol.* 53:420, 1976.

24. Machado-Salas, J., Scheibel, M.E., and Scheibel, A.B. Neuronal changes in the aging mouse: Spinal cord and lower brain stem. *Exp. Neurol.* 54:504, 1977.

25. Buell, S.J. and Coleman, P.D. Dendritic growth in the aged human brain and failure of growth in senile dementia. *Science* 205:854, 1979.

26. Mehraein, P., Yamada, M., and Tarnowska-Dziduszko, E. Quantitative study on dendrites and dentritic spines in Alzheimer's disease and senile dementia. *Adv. Neurol.* 12:453, 1975.

27. Gajdusek, D.C. Unconventional viruses and the origin and disappearance of Kuru. Nobel Lecture. *Science* 197:943, 1977.

28. De Boni, U. and Crapper, D.R. Paired helical filaments of the Alzheimer type in cultured neurones. *Nature* (Lond) 271:566, 1978.

29. Wisniewski, H.M., Bruce, M.E., and Fraser, H. Infectious etiology of neuritic (senile) plaques in mice. *Science* 190:1108, 1975.

27

Pathogenesis of Bacterial Pneumonia in the Elderly: The Effects of Normal Aging Processes

David W. Bentley, M.D.

Pneumonia, in a young or old host, occurs when normal defense mechanisms of the lung are overwhelmed or impaired. Although associated diseases and conditions that more commonly afflict the elderly can play a role [1], the normal aging process per se adversely affects these defense mechanisms. Unfortunately, there are very few studies that have examined this question [2]. The purpose of this report is to review how the normal aging processes might adversely affect the pulmonary defense mechanisms and to stimulate interest in much needed research in this important area.

First I want to consider how two factors, oropharyngeal colonization and "silent" aspiration, predispose the elderly to aspiration of bacteria-laden oropharyngeal secretions and then discuss how the effects of aging might impair the clearance of these secretions.

Oropharyngeal Colonization

Oropharyngeal colonization with bacterial pathogens is a prerequisite for pneumonia in the elderly secondary to aspiration of oropharyngeal secretions. To determine the prevalence of oropharyngeal colonization with gram-negative bacilli in elderly persons with different severities of illness, we performed a cross-sectional survey of 407 volunteers, 65 years of age or older, who had not received antimicrobials in the previous four weeks [3]. Using a single, standardized, throat-culture technique plus a selective-enrichment broth, we noted that gram-negative bacilli were isolated from the oropharynx of relatively healthy elderly subjects in 19% of those living independently in apartments, 23% of residents of a private proprietary home for adults, and 42% of ambulatory residents in health-related facilities. This contrasted with the 8% frequency of colonization in younger individuals (personnel who worked in our hospital and served as controls). Colonization was the highest (60%) in patients on the acute hospital ward of our institution; all had multisystem diseases and several were moribund. The trend of increasing colonization from independent apartments to the acute hospital ward was highly significant ($p < 0.0001$).

The presence of cardiac, respiratory and neoplastic diseases was significantly ($p < 0.05$) associated with colonization, but only if they limited the patient's physical activity or ability to do self care. Also associated with colonization were bladder incontinence, deteriorating or terminal clinical status, inability to ambulate without assistance, and difficulty in performing activities of daily living. Analysis of the independent contribution of each factor to colonization demonstrated that respiratory disease and being bedridden appeared to contribute the most to colonization. Gram-negative bacilli were found in high numbers in the oropharynx of this population; positive throat cultures on direct plating had moderate to heavy growth of gram-negative bacilli in 79% of the specimens.

Previous studies have demonstrated that gram-negative bacilli infrequently colonize the mouth of normal healthy persons apparently due to their poor capacity for attaching to oral surfaces [4] and highly effective clearance mechanisms [5]. The increased frequency and large numbers of gram-negative bacilli in the oropharynx of the institutionalized elderly (especially in the healthy ambulatory residents) suggests that several factors can promote colonization in this population. Factors enhancing attachment and/or adversely affecting the normal clearance mechanisms of the oropharynx might include poor oral hygiene with increased numbers of gram-negative bacilli present in the saliva, decreased flow of saliva and swallowing, decreased desquamation of epithelial cells, diminished salivary glycoproteins or altered epithelial surface glycoproteins [6] and diminished or ineffective secretory (salivary) IgA antibodies [7].

Decreased flow of saliva and decreased swallowing occur during periods of sleep or inactivity and are frequently observed in patients with a bed-to-chair or bedridden existence [8]. I could find no data, however, on any of these factors in the healthy elderly. These studies and studies to determine factors affecting colonization by other respiratory pathogens (especially *s. penumoniae*) in community-based and institution-based elderly populations are needed.

Aspiration of Oropharyngeal Secretions

Bacterial pneumonia in the elderly occurs most commonly from aspiration of oropharyngeal secretions containing bacteria colonizing the naso-oropharynx. Recently, Huxley and colleagues [9] have demonstrated that "silent" aspiration of oropharyngeal contents occurs during sleep in normal persons and even more frequently in subjects with depressed consciousness. By positioning a flexible plastic catheter in the midposterior portion of the nasopharynx and carefully instilling a buffered solution of indium[111] chloride over several hours during the night while the subject slept, they noted the next morning that 45% (9/20) of normal subjects had aspirated into their lungs. There was no correlation with the subjects' age, sex, history of smoking, or previous pneumonia. Aspiration occurred more frequently (70%) and more extensively in the patients with depressed consciousness.

Apparently, normal adults are consistently contaminating their lower respiratory tract with bacteria. Pneumonia, however, is remarkably infrequent because the bacteria in aspirated secretions are usually cleared efficiently by the pulmonary defense mechanisms. Pneumonia develops only when these mechanisms are overwhelmed or impaired, and the aspirated bacteria can rapidly multiply. Presumably, silent aspiration occurs frequently in the elderly but these bacteria-laden secretions are not cleared efficiently. Confirmation of this and the pathophysiologic mechanisms involved require additional studies.

Pulmonary Defense Mechanisms

How might the normal aging processes impair the clearance of these secretions and bacteria? Table 27-1 lists the basic components of man's pulmonary defense system. Time does not permit even a brief review of this system; for this the reader is referred to recent reviews [10,13]. Instead, I will discuss one aspect for which there is data on the effects of aging (mucociliary "elevator") and then discuss some other components (cough reflex, resident alveolar macrophages, humoral immunity, and cell-mediated immunity) where observations are available but for which there is little or no data on the effects of aging.

Table 27-1
Components of the Pulmonary Defense System

Excretory Transport System
Cough reflex**
Mucociliary "elevator"*
Mechanical transport system of alveoli
Lymphohematogenous drainage

Cellular Defenses
Alveolar macrophages (resident)*
Lymphocytes (T and B cells) and the bronchus-associated lymphoid
    tissue (BALT)
Blood monocytes
Blood polymorphs, eosinophiles

Immunologic Defenses
Humoral (secretory) antibody system**
    IgA, IgG, IgE, (C′) (and blood IgM in inflammation)
Cell-mediated immune system**
    T lymphocytes
    Macrophages (and blood monocytes)

Adapted from Johnson et al. [11] with permission of The Johns
Hopkins University Press
*adversely affected by aging
**? adversely affected by aging

Cough Reflex

The cough reflex provides an important mechanism by which excess secretions and bacteria in the trachea or major bronchi can be removed and disposed of by expectoration or swallowing. Although the cough reflex is said to be impaired in old age [1], I could find no studies to support (or deny) this notion. There are, however, a number of well-known effects of normal aging on the lung that can decrease the effectiveness of the cough and lead to retained aspirated bacteria-laden secretions [14].

The diaphragm and accessory muscles for respiration steadily lose strength and effectiveness with age. Intrapulmonary airways seem to be more compliant or "floppy" with age and are more prone to collapse during forced expiration. Airway patency is also reduced as a result of a progressive loss of lung recoil capacity, which leads to decreased maximum expiratory flow rates. The lung parenchyma is affected by a progressive increase in airway closure and closing volume in the lung bases, especially during recumbency, which leads to increased residual volume and decreased vital capacity. These adverse effects of aging on respiratory function lead to an inefficient cough (similar though not as impaired as seen in chronic bronchitis, emphysema, or cystic fibrosis) that can result in retained secretions and even retrograde movement of secretions to the lung periphery or aspiration from one lung to another. This is an important area for future investigations in the elderly.

Mucociliary Transport

The mucociliary "elevator" transport system depends on a morphologically and functionally intact ciliated epithelium as well as normal rheologic properties [15] of respiratory secretions. Ciliated epithelium, mucous glands, and goblet cells extend from the proximal trachea to the terminal bronchioles; the precise life span for the various cell types has not been established. Normally, mechanical clearing of the tracheobronchial tree is a very rapid event with clearance and/or transport rates of 10 mms to 20 mms per min, although rates are slower in the peripheral airways.

Goodman and coworkers [16] have recently investigated the effect of aging on mucociliary function in normal nonsmokers. Mucous transport in the trachea was measured by following with a fluroscopic image intensifier the motion of radioopaque teflon discs blown through the inner channel of a bronchofiberscope. Figure 27-1 summarizes their results. Seven healthy elderly subjects (two men, five women, aged 56 to 70 years, with no recent history of respiratory infection or cough) were compared with ten young healthy subjects (ten men, eight women, aged 19 to 28 years). Mean tracheal mucous velocity in the elderly was significantly slower than in young subjects ($p < 0.05$). Because the discs

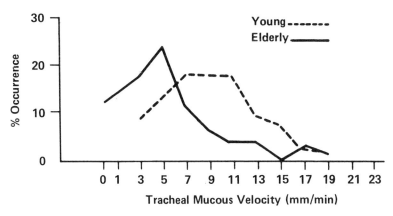

	NO.	RANGE (mm/min)	MEAN±S.D.
YOUNG	10	6.4 –18.8	10.1±3.5
ELDERLY	7	2.3-10.3	5.8±2.6

Figure 27-1. Age comparison of tracheal mucous velocity in young and elderly nonsmokers. Adapted from Goodman et al. [16] with permission of *Am. Rev. Resp. Dis.*

did not travel at uniform velocities in the mucous stream, the frequency histogram was constructed, which included all the disc velocities of every subject in each group. Approximately 10% of all deposited discs in the elderly subjects failed to show a movement at all, whereas all discs in the young subjects showed cephalad motion. There was no consistent differences in pulmonary function for subjects with the fastest and slowest velocities.

Mucociliary transport can be impaired by either one or both of the following: 1) structural and/or functional changes of the cilia or 2) abnormalities in the amount, distribution, and rheologic properties of mucous [15]. I could find no studies, however, on the effect of aging on the function and/or properties of cilia or mucous, respectively. Normally, single or multiple coughs can compensate for decreased transport rates. If, however, a diminished mucociliary transport apparatus plus an ineffective cough mechanism were present in the elderly, important amounts of bacteria-laden secretions would be retained at the terminal bronchial level. If these secretions were not cleared within 3 to 4 hours by these mechanical means, then multiplication of bacteria could occur in the mucous at the alveolar membrane level.

Resident Alveolar Macrophages

Alveolar macrophages are the principal phagocytic cells of the lung [10-13]. As part of the nonspecific, nonimmunologic mechanisms, they can easily phagocytize and kill saprophytic benign commensals that reach the alveolus. More pathogenic bacteria, such as *S. pneumoniae* or *H. influenzae,* are better controlled with the help of opsonins of the IgG class. Alveolar macrophages represent a final effector pathway for not only nonspecific cellular phagocytic defenses but also for specifically triggered cell-mediated immunity via sensitized lymphocytes. In this system, specifically sensitized lymphocytes, following stimulation by specific antigens presented by macrophages, produce a set of biologically active materials (lymphokines) that modulate macrophage function, for example, activation, trapping, and localization of macrophages. Macrophages, stimulated by these antigen-specific mechanisms generally show a nonspecific enhancement for intracellular killing of microorganisms, which is required for intracellular pathogens such as *Listeria monocytogenes* and *M. tuberculosis.*

Despite their principal role, I could find no studies that have specifically examined the quantitative and/or qualitative aspects of alveolar macrophages from elderly human subjects. Are there any conditions that impair the phagocytic activity of pulmonary macrophages that are also frequently present in the healthy elderly? One such condition is hypoxia which, in mice, can depress the in vivo intrapulmonary bacterial killing of inhaled *S. aureus* but has no significant effect on the clearance of *Proteus mirabilis* [17]. Thus, it is not clear how important hypoxia is in impairing bactericidal function of alveolar macrophages.

We do know that hypoxia is one of the results of the normal aging processes of the lung. As noted previously, progressive decrease in lung elastic recoil leads to a decrease in the patency of intrabronchial airways with increased airway closure and closing volume in the lung bases. Because pulmonary blood flow continues to favor the capillaries of the lower zones, there is a disproportion between ventilation and perfusion in the lung bases with an increased alveolar-arterial oxygen gradient and decreased arterial oxygen tension. Sorbini and colleagues [18] noted that arterial oxygen tension declines linearly with age and reaches a mean of 75 mm mercury in the seventh decade. This base-line hypoxia in the normal elderly will increase with any additional causes in regional alveolar hypoventilation and increased inequality of the ventilation-perfusion ratio, for .example, atelectasis secondary to retained secretions. Thus, the stress of hypoxia on pulmonary alveolar macrophages, as noted in animal studies, can play a similar role in the elderly. Because pulmonary antibacterial activities depends largely on the bactericidal activity of the alveolar macrophages, we should investigate carefully alveolar macrophages from elderly human subjects in our studies on the adverse effects of aging on pulmonary clearance.

Humoral Immunity

The immunologic-specific defense mechanisms of the lung consist of local anti-body production (humoral immunity) and cell-mediated immunity [12]. Local humoral immunity in the respiratory tract depends on the local production of adequate concentration and proper function of secretory immunoglobulins. Their role in the pulmonary defense system against bacterial pneumonias is incompletely understood, but they can assist by decreasing attachment of bacteria to mucosa surfaces (IgA), opsonizing bacteria, activating complement, and lysing gram-negative bacilli in the presence of complement (IgG and IgM). The effect of aging on local antibacterial humoral immunity of respiratory mucosa has not been studied.

Aging affects the *systemic* humoral antibody system in several ways [19]. The numbers of immunoglobulin synthesizing plasma cells and concentrations of IgG and IgA are increased. B-cell functions are decreased but many, including decreased circulating heteroantibodies following primary response and increased autoantibodies, are the result of decreased regulatory function of T cells. T-cell independent antibody responses to bacterial and viral vaccines, however, are normal. There are no deficiencies in serum opsonic activity or functional assays for the classical complement or alternate complement pathways.

It is not clear what role (if any) cell-mediated immunity plays in increasing the host's resistance to pyogenic bacteria that commonly cause bacterial pneumonia in the elderly. The notion that cell-mediated immunity can play a role is appealing, however, because aging affects primarily the cell-mediated immune system [19].

Decreased thymic lymphocyte mass and germinal centers are commonly noted. In addition there is a marked decrease in vitro in the capacity of T cells to respond to antigens, and decreased antibody response to T-cell-dependent antigens has been demonstrated. In vivo studies reveal decreased delayed hyper-sensitivity response to skin testing antigens. It is important to note that there is a good correlation between local cell-mediated immunity (migration inhibition factor produced by sensitized lymphocytes) and systemic delayed dermal hyper-sensitivity to the same immunizing antigen following bacterial infection of the lower respiratory tract. The role of cell-mediated immunity in the elderly's response to bacterial pneumonia can prove a fruitful area for investigation.

Recently Phair and colleagues [20] compared host defense mechanisms of hospitalized patients older than age 60 to those of younger hospitalized patients and to nonhospitalized controls to determine if altered defense mechanisms could be correlated with nosocomial carriage of pathogens and the development of hospital-acquired pneumonia. Although a number of alterations were noted in the elderly, none were significantly different from the younger age group, and there was no significant correlation with colonization and/or pneumonia.

Summary

The pathogenesis of bacterial pneumonia in the elderly remains unclear. We know that oropharyngeal colonization with respiratory pathogens is a prerequisite for pneumonia in the elderly secondary to aspiration of oropharyngeal secretions. One study indicates that gram-negative bacilli frequently (and in large numbers) colonize the oropharynx of the elderly. A number of factors that promote increased adherence of other major respiratory pathogens, such as *S. pneumoniae* and *S. aureus,* can exist in the oropharynx of the elderly. Silent aspiration of bacteria-laden oropharyngeal secretions can occur more frequently in the elderly. In the presence of an ineffective cough and decreased mucociliary transport mechanisms, these bacteria-laden oropharyngeal secretions would be retained long enough for multiplication of large numbers of bacteria in the mucous. The normally lowered arterial oxygen tension seen with aging plus any additional increases in hypoxia secondary to retained secretions can further impair alveolar macrophage function. In addition, alveolar macrophages can sustain adverse metabolic and/or immunologic changes as a result of aging per se. The role of impaired T-cell function, a characteristic feature of the normal immunologic processes in the elderly, is unclear but may be important.

Study of the pathogenesis of bacterial pneumonia in the elderly is a rewarding area for research from which intervention efforts can then logically proceed. We need the interest and skills of our best researchers to achieve these goals.

References

1. Freeman, E. The respiratory system. In J.C. Brocklehurst, *Textbook of Geriatric Medicine and Gerontology.* Edinburgh-London-New York: Churchill Livingstone, 1978.

2. Phair, J.P., Kauffman, C.A. and Bjornson, A. Investigation of host defense mechanisms in the aged as determinants of nosocomial colonization and pneumonia. *J. Reticuloendothel. Soc.* 23:397, 1978.

3. Valenti, W.M., Trudell, R.G., and Bentley D.W. Factors predisposing to oropharyngeal colonization with gram-negative bacilli in the aged. *N. Engl. J. Med.* 298:1108, 1978.

4. Ellen, R.P. and Gibbons, R.J. Parameters affecting the adherence and tissue tropisms of *Streptococcus pygenes. Infect Immunity* 9:85, 1974.

5. LaForce, F.M., Hopkins, J., Trow, R., et al. Human oral defenses against gram-negative rods. *Am. Rev. Respir. Dis.* 114:929, 1975.

6. Williams, R.C. and Gibbons, R.J. Inhibition of streptococcal attachment to receptors on human buccal epithelial cells by antigenically similar salivary glycoproteins. *Infect. Immun.* 11:711, 1975.

7. Gibbons, R.J. Bacterial adherence to mucosal surfaces and its inhibi-

tion by secretory antibodies. In J. Mestecky and A.R. Lawton (Eds.), *The Immunoglobulin A System.* New York: Plenum Publishing Corp., 1974.

8. Lear, C.S.C., Flanagan, J.B., Jr., and Moorrees, C.E.A. The frequency of deglutition in man. *Arch. Oral. Biol.* 10:83, 1965.

9. Huxley, E.J., Vroslav, J., Gray, W.R., and Pierce, A.K., Pharyngeal aspiration in normal adults and patients with depressed consciousness. *Am. J. Med.* 64:564, 1978.

10. Green, G.M., Jakab, G.J., Low, R.B., et al. State of the art: Defense mechanisms of the respiratory membrane. *Am. Rev. Resp. Dis.* 115:479, 1977.

11. Johnson, III J.R., and Phillip, J.R. The defense of the lung: Studies of the role of cell-mediated immunity. *The Johns Hopkins Med. J.* 141:126, 1977.

12. Kaltreider, H.B. State of the art: Expression of immune mechanisms in the lung. *Am. Rev. Resp. Dis.* 113:347, 1976.

13. Turner-Warwick, M. *Immunology of the Lung.* Chicago: Year Book Med. Publ. Inc., 1978.

14. Campbell, E.J., and Lefrak, S.S. How aging affects the structure and function of the respiratory system. *Geriat.* 33(6):68, 1978.

15. Wanner, A. State of the art: Clinical aspects of mucociliary transport. *Am. Rev. Resp. Dis.* 116:73, 1977.

16. Goodman, R.M., Yergin, B.M., et al. Relationship of smoking history and pulmonary function tests to tracheal mucous velocity in non-smokers, young smokers, ex-smokers, and patients with chronic bronchitis. *Am. Rev. Resp. Dis.* 117:205, 1978.

17. Green, G.M., and Kass, E.H. The influence of bacterial species on pulmonary resistance to infection in mice subjected to hypoxia, cold stress, and ethanolic intoxication. *Brit. J. Exptl. Pathol.* 46:360, 1965.

18. Sorbini, C.A., Grassi, V., Solinas, E., et al. Arterial oxygen tension in relation to age in healthy subjects. *Resp.* 25:3, 1968.

19. Makinodan, T. Immunity and aging. In T. Makinodan (Ed.) *Handbook of the Biology of Aging.* New York: Van Nostrand Reinhold Co., 1977.

20. Phair, J.P., Kauffman, C.A., and Bjornson, A. Investigation of host defense mechanisms in the aged as determinants of nosocomial colonization and pneumonia. *J. Reticuloendothel. Soc.* 23:397, 1978.

28 The Role of Health Services Research in Geriatrics

Robert L. Kane, M.D.

As geriatrics emerges as a discipline in its own right, a solid research network must be developed. As geriatrics matures into a practice field, mechanisms for gathering, maintaining, and utilizing knowledge must be put in place. Research is a critical component of a geriatric program.

Currently, our understanding of the aging process and its attendant illnesses and health-care needs are merely in embryonic stages, despite numerous opportunities to accumulate data. If the currently available data were assembled into a useable body of knowledge, health-care providers could make more confident predictions about the effects of their ministrations on the physical, psychological, and social status of their patients.

The first cohorts of academic geriatricians in the United States have a major obligation to begin this research process. If geriatrics is to become an academic discipline to prepare a new generation of geriatric specialists or to educate generalist physicians who are sensitive to the needs of the aged, tactics by which a neophyte geriatrician can proficiently accumulate, process, and regenerate information need to be established [15].

There is no scarcity of research opportunities. A number of reviews and agendas for research in biomedical and social science areas have been offered [1,2,4,10,21]. Rather than repeat them here I will address the needs and opportunities for research on the problems of delivering health-care services to older persons and the ways by which health services research can contribute to a program of geriatric education.

A number of critical areas must be investigated by a health services research program. Measurement tools used to define the patient's health status need to be refined and clarified, not only for effectiveness in obtaining a clear picture of existing status, but for making predictions for future care. We must consider the possibility that geriatrics requires a new taxonomy more suited to the patient with multiple problems than is the prevalent diagnostic nomenclature. Effectiveness and relevancy of existing health-care procedures experienced by geriatric patients must be evaluated, giving iatrogenesis more than a cursory glance. Clinical epidemiology can be used to establish norms for the geriatric population and to permit the development of prognostic indicators. Health services research is necessary not only for the practitioner to see how services are utilized but how key health-related decisions about elderly patients are made. Additionally, the cost effectiveness of different modes of care must be addressed. Furthermore, we must also examine the value preferences that the elderly themselves use in making health-related decisions.

Measures

A prerequisite to geriatric health-care services research is refinement of the methods for assessing and measuring the status of elderly persons. Obviously, those delivering medical care to the elderly need technical knowledge and skill derived from the medical specialties relevant to the treating of particular problems. Beyond that they require a general perception about the well-being of the older person that transcends a particular diagnosis, problem, or specialization. Many authorities have pointed to the limitations of a diagnosis-centered approach to the health care of the elderly [8,17,26]. Conventional wisdom now holds that: 1) the elderly are subject to multiple diagnoses; 2) the physical, mental, and social well-being of an elderly individual are very closely interrelated, so that multidimensional assessments of health status are necessary; and 3) assessment tools that examine the ability to function independently despite disease, physical and mental disability, and social deprivation are the most useful overall indicators to assist those caring for the elderly.

Although current literature is replete with correlative studies reporting the relationship of demographic and other variables to the health status of the elderly, there is a shortage of studies that truly represent a history of an elderly person. Those existing studies are valuable, but they fall short because the data are often presented with insufficient reference to the measurements on which the statements are based.

Recent reviews of measurements in long-term care [3] or of classes of measurements, such as those of functional status [7,16], of subjective well-being or happiness [6,18], of life adjustment [9], and of mental functioning or depression [5,22,23,24], indicate that measures are numerous but are often not thoroughly tested. In some instances, measurement tools that were created for different age groups and specific problems unrelated to an aging patient (for example, tests for psychiatric patients) are being applied to the elderly. In other instances, rather than using an evaluation test that has been fielded with an elderly population, an entirely new instrument will be developed, with no real reason for doing so. Developmental work to produce valid testing instruments requires that each component be evaluated and that the entire instrument be tested for accuracy, validity, reproducibility, and reliability.

The development of measurements requires the participation of psychometricians. Such personnel can be attached to geriatric units so that the developmental work will proceed within the context of long-term care. Although physicians would not be expected to perform the bulk of this initial work, they will have important contributions to make. The evaluation of the impact of programs requires these tools as well as the monitoring of outcomes of specific therapies. Furthermore, before the interaction of physical, mental, and social outcomes can be studied, each construct must be amenable to separate measurement.

Effectiveness of Care

Once measurement capability has been established, geriatricians can begin to examine the effectiveness of clinical regimens and various patterns of care delivery. The investigators would have the opportunity to show empirically to what extent the overall goals of long-term care (survival, independence, contentment, freedom from discomfort, mental alertness) are compatible with each other and to what extent tradeoffs are necessary.

The other side of effectiveness is iatrogenesis, which deserves investigation as an important research topic. The elderly receive a disproportionate amount of diagnosis and treatment compared with younger patients. One would, therefore, expect them to be vulnerable to a commensurate number of iatrogenic complications. We need to know to what extent medical interventions lead to a deterioration in the patient's status. Geriatricians emphasize the delicate equilibrium of the elderly patient, who is frequently unable to handle additional physical or emotional insults. Much of medical care can be described as a prime source of assaults on both psyche and soma. Test populations of elderly persons, stratified to encompass common diagnoses and a wide range of functional status, need to be structured to assess what number of episodes of sudden decline in health status are associated with medical procedures, such as drugs, treatments, or surgery. The risk/benefit ratio for therapy, a parameter at least considered in younger persons but rarely in the elderly, needs to be studied.

Although medical interventions for the elderly can be dangerous (adverse drug reactions, for example, occur more frequently than in younger people), it is uncertain whether these reactions are due to inherent susceptibility or poor compliance (perhaps produced by a combination of decreased memory and complex regimens). A useful series of studies could be designed to determine whether medical iatrogenesis is a major or a minor element in the overall health picture of the elderly and what proportion of it is attributable to patterns of care or other provider characteristics. Models for experiments in related areas are available to aid in the design of such studies [12].

A more subtle dimension of the iatrogenesis question concerns the effects of the general patient-management decisions made by geriatric providers. Elderly persons have been known to manifest marked losses in functional ability, including declines in mental status, when moved to an unfamiliar environment.

Seligman has termed this phenomenon of withdrawal and apathy among institutionalized individuals "learned helplessness" [25]. Disorientation is likely to be greater in unfamiliar surroundings. Rigid routines can leave the patient with aggressive, sometimes even abusive, behavior as the only means of self-expression. If referral to a nursing home is made as part of a recuperative process, this, as well as any drug or surgical procedure involved, might contribute to functional decline. This emotionally charged issue should be objectively studied.

Clinical Epidemiology

Many of the issues relevant to geriatric practice can be approached from an epidemiologic perspective. We might begin with a very basic question: what problems account for most of the hospital admissions among the elderly or for most long-term-care days? The cursory data available suggest that a few common problems account for a substantial proportion of patient difficulties. For example, the most frequent causes for admission to geriatric wards in Britiain are falls, strokes, incontinence, and mental confusion [11]. These causes present us with multiple research opportunities in both clinical research and health services research. The clinical researcher might study cardiac arrhythmias that affect cerebral blood flow or explore problems in proprioception and balance. The health services researcher might investigate how the organization of services and the service delivery environment exacerbate or ameliorate these problems. We have already noted the likelihood that many treatments and procedures are not necessary. Similarly, the routines of the short-stay hospital may need altering for the elderly. Three weeks without being dressed and allowed out of bed can seriously affect the functional abilities of the elderly. Geriatricians need to develop information about social and environmental factors correlated with the incidence and prevalence of common geriatric problems.

Research into these common problems of geriatrics offers an opportunity to combine the interests of the clinician and the health services researcher. For example, how can we identify those individuals at greatest risk of suffering from falls (or incontinence)? What are the circumstances associated with these untoward events in terms of physiologic phenomena (arrhythmias or hypotension in the case of falls), activities, and precipitating events? Settings such as the Veterans Administration hospitals offer an excellent opportunity for this type of research (although generalization is difficult because of the special characterization of the male population served). However, the large identifiable and traceable population greatly facilitates prospective studies. Also, long-term follow-up is feasible, which permits analysis of patterns of recurrence and comparison of treatment goals with actual outcomes. Treated groups can be compared with untreated or alternatively treated controls.

Toward Prognostic Indicators

Once outcome measures are clearly established, controlled clinical trials of various methods of managing elderly patients can be fielded and the effects measured in terms of physical, mental, and social functioning. Such trials are appropriate when genuine doubt exists about the relative merits of alternative approaches to achieve an outcome that is clearly valued by the patient population. It is worthwhile, for example, to test the ability of geriatric assessment units to maximize the patient's possibility of returning to the community or the extent to which geriatric day-hospital attendance is associated with improved functional status. For studies such as these, randomized assignment to various experimental (and control) conditions is both sorely needed and ethically justified when resources are scarce so that there are more candidates for geriatric assessment units or day hospitals than could presently be served, and the effects of the care are uncertain. If care in specialized geriatric units was associated with decreased independence or well-being, one would not wish to encourage a continuation of such care services. Similarly, controlled clinical trials can be used to test the marginal benefits of increments of service, such as adding home visits of occupational therapists or adding counseling services.

Many times, however, controlled clinical trials are not appropriate for ethical or logistic reasons. For example, in settings where it is impractical or politically unacceptable to give two distinct types of care, then the effect of services can be judged only in comparison with some reasonable prognosis of outcome for the particular case. This suggests a line of research directed at establishing average prognoses for conditions common to the elderly. (Although this technique is applicable to chronic disease in general, it has special relevance for the elderly where advanced age can be an important factor.) Prognoses for long-term-care patients with varying conditions must be established along the dimensions of all the important goals of geriatric care. Such work is a laborious but inescapable methodologic requirement for further studies of the elderly because it provides a basis for comparing outcomes of alternative treatment when randomized trials are not feasible.

In brief, elderly patients must first be classified according to a well-organized system of diagnosis and staging. Then a team of experts could make prognostic estimations related to goals of care, using temporal targets (such as 3 months, 6 months, or 1 year). The actual health status of each patient can be determined at each agreed-upon point and compared with the original prognosis. Ultimately, when a set of reliable prognoses has been determined, these can be recorded and codified. Mathematical modeling (for example, discriminate analysis and regression) can be used to identify those factors most useful in prediction. Such a process would be repeated until a sufficiently high level of predictive accuracy is achieved. The goal is to reduce such predictions to average prognostic statements, which can be applied to various populations with defined characteristics. Numerous iterations are needed to produce workable formulae for estimating such averages.

The result of these efforts is equivalent to a natural history for a group of patients with specified characteristics. This information provides a probability estimate of the role of change from one status to another, an estimate that offers a critical contribution to any efforts to describe decision-trees for patient care [13]. Decision analysis of this type requires a careful specification of the decisions to be made and the alternative outcomes that result from each decision. The product of the probability of an event (an outcome) times the value of that event yields a net value that can be summed for each branch of the tree.

Once available, average prognoses can be readily applied in many other studies as well. For example, they can be used to determine whether monetary or other incentives to caretakers can lead to better outcomes than the standard prognoses. Another use would be to compare the cost and effectiveness of various configurations of health-care personnel. Two existing studies have indicated that geriatric nurse practitioners working with a physician can provide satisfactory primary care in nursing homes [14,20]. In one of these studies, a social worker also made a significant contribution to the outcome [14]. In neither study, however, were medical, psychological, or functional outcomes estimated and compared with a suitable control population of known average prognosis. Patients were not classified according to levels of necessary care nor were several permutations of team health care assessed. Thus, much remains to be done before these crucial questions can be answered.

Similarly, studies are needed comparing effectiveness and cost of various configurations of living conditions and health-care settings. Alternatives to nursing home placement (home care, home-care-plus-day-care centers, residential communities with specialized services available) are frequently proposed. A recent controversial study suggests, however, that such plans can be significantly more expensive than nursing home care [27]. Are they correspondingly more effective than nursing home care? We could rephrase this question to ask whether the average outcome is better than standard prognoses for patients in various levels of initial status. The experimental design to address the restated question is more readily apparent.

A major development in the field of long-term care is the growing emphasis on case management. Data from the GAO study in Cleveland have suggested that it is possible to classify both the care needed by and the services rendered to a population of elderly individuals. These can then be combined in a matrix that compares level of need and services received. Further analyses can calculate the rate of change over time that can, in turn, be related to the care received [19, 28]. This study utilized a taxonomy of services rendered that was sufficiently encompassing to include a wide variety of medical and social services. Longer periods of follow-up would permit more precise calculations of the probabilities of an elderly individual's going from one status to another.

Education for Research

The brief list of examples noted here of health services research opportunities in geriatrics illustrates the variety of projects that might be undertaken to answer questions important to the development of the field. If such research is to be carried out under the auspices of geriatric units, attention in the geriatric curriculum must be given to the preparation of geriatric researchers. Although geriatrics is very much an interdisciplinary enterprise in research as well as in practice, the role of properly prepared physicians is critical to both. The training of geriatricians in the performance of health services research can be accomplished at both formal and informal levels. Basic background research design and statistical principles (including measurement) is best acquired through classroom work, or at least formally structured learning experiences, but, as with clinical practice, there is no substitute for direct application of the formally acquired skills.

A teaching unit in geriatrics should have one or more active health services research projects. These projects become the training wards of the geriatrician at various stages of development. As in the case of clinical training, the student can participate at a level appropriate to acquired skills—from a data collector to a designer and analyst. Through an apprenticeship with an ongoing research project, a medical student can develop skills in defining aspects of geriatric care more precisely as well as an appreciation for the problems of measuring relevant parameters. A geriatric fellow can utilize the opportunity to develop a personal research protocol on a topic of particular interest. Even if the fellow's career plans are not directed toward academics, new insights will be gained into the management of geriatric patients.

It is unnecessary to belabor the role of research in enhancing the position and prestige of geriatrics within the academic milieu. An active research program represents a commitment to scholarship that is essential to academic growth. What may be less readily appreciable is the contribution health services research can make to clinical care. Especially in an actively developing area like geriatrics, the discipline of formulating researchable questions, translating those into measurable elements, and assessing the results of intervention can provide new insights and rigor for practice. The ability of geriatrics to define meaningful areas of inquiry, to develop new strategies to improve the care for the elderly, and to offer new formulations of the problems encountered will be critical in establishing its image in the eyes of students, colleagues, and the general public.

References

1. Binstock, R.H. and Shanas, E. (Eds.). *Handbook of Aging and the Social Sciences*. New York: Van Nostrand Reinhold Company, 1976.
2. Birren, J.E. and Schaie, K.W. (Eds.). *Handbook of the Psychology of Aging*. New York: Van Nostrand Reinhold Company, 1977.
3. Bloom, M. Evaluation instruments: Tests and measurements in long-term care. In S. Sherwood (Ed.) *Long-Term Care: A Handbook for Researchers, Planners and Providers*. New York: Spectrum, 1975.
4. Finch, C.E. and Hayflick, L. (Eds.). *Handbook of the Biology of Aging*. New York: Van Nostrand Reinhold Company, 1977.
5. Gallagher, D., Thompson, L.W., and Levy, S.M. Clinical psychological assessment of older adults. In L. Poor (Ed.) *Aging in the 1980's: Selected Contemporary Issues in the Psychology of Aging*. Washington, D.C.: American Psychological Association, 1980.
6. George, L.K. The happiness syndrome: Methodological and substantive issues in the study of social psychological well-being in adulthood. *Gerontologist* 19:210, 1979.
7. Goga, J.A. and Hambacher, W.D. Psychologic and behavioral assessment of geriatric patients: A review. *J. Am. Geriatr. Soc.* 25:232, 1977.
8. Goran, M., Crystal, R., Ford, L., and Tebbutt, J. PSRO review of LTC utilization and quality. *Med. Care* 14:94, 1976.
9. Graney, M.J. and Graney, E.E. Scaling adjustment in older people. *Int. J. Aging Hum. Dev.* 4:351, 1973.
10. Institute of Medicine. *Aging and Medical Education*. Washington, D.C.: National Academy of Sciences, 1978.
11. Isaacs, B., Livingston, M., and Neville, Y. *Survival of the Unfittest: A Study of Geriatric Patients in Glasgow*. London: Routledge & Kegan Paul, 1972.
12. Jick, H. The discovery of drug-induced illness. *N. Engl. J. Med.* 296, 1977.
13. Kane, H.L. and Kane, R.A. Alternatives to institutional care of the elderly: Beyond the dichotomy. *The Gerontologist* (in press).
14. Kane, R.L., Jorgensen, L.A., Teteberg, B., and Kuwahara, J. Is good nursing-home care feasible? *JAMA* 235:516, 1976.
15. Kane, R.L., Solomon, D.H., Beck, J.C., Keeler, E., and Kane, R.A. *Geriatrics in the United States: Manpower Projections and Training Considerations*. R-2543-HJK. Santa Monica, Calif.: The Rand Corporation, 1980.
16. Katz, S., Hedrick, S. and Henderson, N. The measurement of long-term care needs and impact. *Health and Medical Care Services Review* 2:2, 1979.
17. Kent, D., Kastenbaum, R., and Sherwood S. (Eds.) *Research Planning and Action for the Elderly*. New York: Behavioral Publications, 1972.
18. Larson, R. Thirty years of research on the subjective well-being of older Americans. *J. Gerontol.* 33:109, 1978.

19. Maddox, G.L. and Dellinger, D.C. Assessment of functional status in a program evaluation and resource allocation model. *Annals of the American Academy of Political and Social Science* 436:59, 1978.

20. Mark, R.G., Willemain, T.R., Malcolm, T., Master, R.J., and Clarkson, T. *Final Report of the Nursing Home Telemedicine Project.* Vol. 1. Washington, D.C.: National Science Foundation, 1976.

21. National Institute on Aging. *Special Report on Aging, 1979.* Publ. No. 79-1907. Washington, D.C.: Government Printing Office, 1979.

22. Raskin, A. and Jarvik, L.F. *Psychiatric Symptoms and Cognitive Loss in the Elderly.* Washington, D.C.: Hemisphere Publishing Corporation, 1979.

23. Salzman, C., Shader, R.T., Kochansky, G.E., and Cronin, D.M. Rating scales for psychotropic drug research with geriatric patients. I. Behavior ratings. *J. Am. Geriatric. Soc.* 20:209, 1972a.

24. Salzman, C., Kochansky, G.E., Shader, R.L. and Cronin, D.M. Rating scales for psychotropic drug research with geriatric patients. II. Mood ratings. *J. Am. Geriatric. Soc.* 20:215, 1972b.

25. Seligman, M. *Helplessness: On Depression, Development and Death.* San Francisco, Calif.: W.H. Freeman and Company, 1975.

26. Sherwood, S. *Long-Term Care: A Handbook for Researchers, Planners and Providers.* New York: Spectrum, 1975.

27. Weissert, W.G., Wan, T.T.H., and Livieratos, B.B., *Effects and Costs of Day Care and Homemaker Services for the Chronically Ill: A Randomized Experiment.* DHEW Publ #(PHS)79-3258. Washington, D.C.: Government Printing Office, 1980.

28. U.S. Comptroller General. *The Well-Being of Older People in Cleveland.* Ohio Publ. No. (HED)77-70. Washington, D.C.: Government Printing Office. 1977.

V
Interprofessional Training in Geriatric Medicine

29 Introduction

Stanley J. Brody, J.D., M.S.W.

The literature of geriatrics and gerontology is replete with acknowledgements that the health problems of the elderly reflect the interrelationships of physical, psychological and social impairments [1]. It is equally agreed that care and support for the elderly are shared by many disciplines and professions, and there is some awareness that the optimum delivery of services requires not only multidisciplinary efforts but interprofessional collaboration as well.

In recognition of the complex needs of elderly patients, educational programs are being developed to provide multiple professions an opportunity to interact in didactic and clinical settings. These require a comprehensive approach utilizing varied disciplinary supports in assessment, treatment, and care. To understand the difficulties that beset such an effort necessitates an acknowledgement of the societal ambience in which it is undertaken.

The critical condition confronting educators is the unequal appreciations by the community of the medical and health/social service interventions. As Engel has put it, scientific medicine is the dogma of western civilization [2] and public appropriations as a mark of societal values have followed that sentiment. The comparative values placed on these two service components is best articulated in the federal budgetary expression of thirty billion dollars for medical care and one billion for health/social services in response to the health needs of the elderly [1]. Even more expressive is the oft heard comment of the aged patient, that "I put myself in the hands of the doctor."

While federal service delivery support has followed this unequal dichotomy between medicine and health/social services, there have been new initiatives taken to interrelate these two main professional foci, at least in the educational field. The first such effort was made by the Veterans Administration through the establishment of geriatric research, education, and clinical care centers, which require multidisciplinary approaches. Additionally, the Institute of Medicine of the National Academy of Sciences Report on Geriatric Medical Education, funded by the National Institute on Aging (NIA), called for educational opportunities in medical schools for interprofessional experience [3]. Grants for the development of a multidisciplinary curriculum in geriatric medical education were authorized by the Health Manpower Administration in 1979. Simultaneously, the Administration on Aging (AoA) offered geriatric fellowship programs emphasizing the multi-medical-specialty mutuality of interest in the aged. The AoA has also funded long-term-care demonstration programs that are keyed to the participation of medical schools. For the last three years, AoA has supported university educational training programs involving the various health professions including medicine.

It is with this background in mind that Rodney Coe, Ph.D. presents a socio-logical perspective outlining the barriers to achieving interprofessional training and recognizing the signs of change that can enable educators to surmount these obstacles. Bess Dana, M.S.S.A. joins in seeing similar possibilities for change in medical education suggesting that geriatric education can present the oppor-tunity to broaden all of medical and social work education. While identifying many of the same barriers as Coe, she outlines a conceptual base for the develop-mental process necessary to achieve interprofessional education.

The experience under the federal rubric of Area Health Education Centers of Morton Rapoport, M.D. and Barbara Cahn, M.S.W. follows. They describe the University of Maryland's efforts to develop an interdisciplinary education and service program and highlight the difficulties inherent in such an enterprise. The issues that Coe and Dana comment on are considered within Maryland's program development with the added involvement of the community. Of particular in-terest from a pragmatic point of view is the resolution of the conflicting time constraints of each of the participating professional schools.

All of the participants in the discussion of these papers emphasize the need to reenforce and acknowledge the contribution made by each of the participat-ing professions. It was generally agreed that no interdisciplinary educational program would be successful unless the identity and validity of the contribution, knowledge, and skill of each discipline was supported by all. Equally important was the unanimity expressed in accepting the clinical component as the key to a successful interprofessional educational experience. Didactic presentations are seen as complementary to yet an integral part of the clinical program.

References

1. Brody, S.J. The thirty-to-one paradox: Health needs of the aged and medical solutions. *National Journal,* Vol II, 44:1869, 1979.

2. Engel, G.L. The need for a new medical model: A challenge for biomedi-cine. *Science* 196:129, 1977.

3. Institute of Medicine. *Aging and Medical Education.* Washington, D.C.: National Academy of Sciences, 1978.

30 A Sociological Perspective

Rodney M. Coe, Ph.D.

The purpose of this chapter is to identify some factors related to current trends in interdisciplinary or interprofessional training in geriatric medicine in the United States. From a perspective on social change, this will involve describing barriers to change as well as new developments that offer possibilities for overcoming the barriers. First, however, it is important to note briefly what we mean by interdisciplinary training and why geriatric care requires interdisciplinary training.

Interprofessional training is the educational preparation of members of different disciplines for the coordinated application of the special skills toward a common goal. In this case, the common goal is comprehensive care for the elderly. Note the definition does not specify which disciplines are included since this may vary from situation to situation. Nor are specific elements of educational preparation named since these may vary in duration, intensity, and degree of integration. However, the definition does imply preservation of the special knowledge and skills of the different disciplines and emphasizes their coordinated application to the needs of the elderly. Educational preparation also implies development of a shared understanding of team goals and appreciation of the roles of other disciplines in achieving those goals.

Given this definition of interprofessional training, it is not difficult to see how it would apply to geriatric medicine. In the first place, the health problems of the elderly extend far beyond the biological dimensions that are most often the focus of treatment by physicians. In fact, because most of the diseases of the elderly are chronic and degenerative in nature, biological interventions alone are of questionable effectiveness. Effective resolution of multifaceted problems requires application of multifaceted skills. Since no one professional group has all the requisite skills and knowledge, an interdisciplinary approach is indicated.

Second, the problem of providing adequate care for the elderly is growing in the sense of an increased proportion of elderly in the population and the rising demand for health-related services. In this census year (1980), it is estimated that there are some 23 million persons age 65 and over who represent about 11 percent of the total population. Demographers have estimated that by 2020, the proportion may exceed 16 percent [1]. More important, the fastest growing segment of the population even now is the age group 75 and over, and this is the group that uses disproportionately more health-related services. It is also well known that elderly average more visits to physicians' offices and use more hospital days of care than younger age groups. Furthermore, health-related problems, especially of the older segment of the elderly population, extend beyond strictly medical concerns to problems such as those of nutrition, transportation, and income.

A third reason why interdisciplinary training is important for geriatric medicine relates to a change in values regarding outcomes in health care for the elderly. Specifically, this refers to the shift from an emphasis on custodial care to rehabilitation for elderly patients. This shift in values has not occurred uniformly in all settings, of course, but more progressive programs have applied the general principles of rehabilitation to problems of the elderly. As is well known, rehabilitation is a process that demands interprofessional collaboration [2].

Problems in Interprofessional Collaboration

Compelling reasons for interprofessional training notwithstanding, there remain several important barriers to the development of a consensus as to the need for such programs and for the implementation of effective training programs in geriatric medicine. In fact, the barriers to interprofessional collaboration (cultural and status differences and ambiguity in role responsibilities) that were described nearly two decades ago [3] still seem to be operative today. Cultural differences among professionals refer primarily to the language of a discipline, its definitions and perspectives. Clearly, substantial differences remain in technical terms relevant to the multifaceted problems of the elderly just as there are differences in whether the perspective is on the individual or on the group.

Status differences reflect variation in power and influence associated with one's place in the social structure. The status hierarchy among health professionals is well-defined and is relatively unchanging, due in part to the historical legacy of how professional groups obtained control of the work of their discipline and how the occupational boundaries are maintained and protected. Tasks related to care of the elderly require the coordination of skills of more than one professional group and, the relative importance of a discipline's expertise can change from one situation to another. Effective coordination requires flexibility in assignment of decision-making roles, and this is difficult to achieve with the present, relatively rigid, status hierarchy.

Finally, role ambiguity refers to lack of understanding of how one's own skills relate to the skills of other members of the interdisciplinary team. Most professional training is conducted along disciplinary lines with only superficial efforts at collaborative education for teamwork or even at understanding what special skills others have that complement one's own. As a consequence, most professionals do not know how to work effectively with members of other professions and tend to fall back on traditional patterns of stratified relationships with other professionals. This is not to say that, over time, experience with others will not result in examples of effective collaboration, because it does happen. But this is a slow and sometimes painful method for achieving a goal that could more effectively be accomplished by establishing interdisciplinary programs early in the training career.

More recent analyses have cited certain characteristics of a profession as a major barrier to interprofessional training and collaboration. The main theme is "professional dominance" of the organization and functioning of health services by medicine [4]. Not only does medicine control its own work—who enters the profession, what standards of training and performance are required, and who is licensed—but, critics claim, medicine also (unduly) controls or influences the work conditions of other health professionals, what services can be provided, how they are to be organized, and how they are to be financed.

A related trend is the broadened definition of health problems—what sociologists call "medicalization of deviance" [5]. This means that behaviors that once were defined as deviant (alcoholism, drug addiction, disability, deformity, and so on) are now defined as illness. Therefore, the responsibility for treatment falls to the medical profession. Increasingly, physicians are called on to give advice or provide treatment for problems for which they have had little or no specific training. Personnel skilled in these health-related matters are often available but are unable to function effectively without the physician's cooperation.

To the extent that this is an accurate description of the power of medicine, it would be its responsibility to initiate and encourage interprofessional collaboration and coordination of services to provide comprehensive care. Most analysts suggest, however, that maintaining the status quo and the dominant position in it is the main concern of the profession [6].

These general criticisms can be seen also in the context of geriatric medicine. An article published in the *Journal of the American Geriatrics Society* [7] reported that practicing physicians are generally reluctant to get involved in the care of the elderly, especially in settings like nursing homes. Furthermore, doctors tend to be unenthusiastic about the routine care of elderly patients for reasons that include the lack of likelihood of cure, a perception of the problems as uninteresting, and even concern about growing old themselves. Just as important, the next generation of practitioners may not be very different since there has been little emphasis or interest in gerontology or geriatrics.

As late as 1976, only 15% of the 96 medical schools responding to a survey taught geriatrics as a separate subject. Eighty-two percent of them considered the chance encounter with elderly patients as training in geriatrics. Only two schools required an experience in geriatrics. The authors concluded that medical schools were continuing to assign low priority to geriatrics and were making little effort to present information relevant to aging and the case of older people in a systematic, coherent manner [8].

Limiting Conditions

Although there seems to be increased efforts both in public and private sectors to address the problems of the elderly—and I will identify some of these efforts—several current trends mitigate against making much progress. Chief among these is the continued trend toward professional differentiation and specialization, both within and among the health professions, in the absence of a complementary effort to increase coordination of the application of specialized professional skills. Continued specialization places limits on the specialist's knowledge of and ability to work with professionals in other disciplines. Practical issues of licensure of allied health practitioners, distribution of specialists and subspecialists in the population, even the continuing costs of professional services, are related to this trend. Furthermore, one study has shown that students in the health professions interested in subspecialties (and this is a majority) have a less-positive attitude toward the elderly than do students interested in primary-care specialties although there were no differences between the groups in amounts of knowledge about the elderly [9].

A related but separate trend is continued uncoordinated operation of independent health-service agencies in the community. We are all familiar with the keen competition among hospitals for the latest technology, the most diversified and capable staff, and the highest occupancy rate. There is also competition among other elements of the system, both public and private. The problem was identified some time ago but efforts to plan for and coordinate use of a community's health resources, such as comprehensive health planning or the current health systems agency programs, have not been successful [10].

Margolis [11] suggested that part of the reason for failure to alter the American health delivery system is that key elements, medicine included, attempt to resolve problems generated by changing disease patterns without changing their own structure. The shift from acute to chronic disease in the past 50 years is well known. Yet we persist in trying to deal with these problems in a system that emphasizes expensive high technology acute care and maintains financing mechanisms that contribute to runaway costs of care and inhibit development of needed coordinated levels of services.

A third major barrier is the relative inflexibility of the processes of medical and other professional education. Although a need for change in medical training has been noted, especially with respect to gerontology and geriatrics, some obstacles remain. These include the existence of an intensive curriculum that is already extensive in time with little room for "new" topics to be added; a departmentalized instruction program that tends to resist integration of subject matter; a decreasing number of personnel who have diminishing financial resources available for the development of new programs; the fact that training is carried on in isolation from other health professional students; and the lack of faculty interest in stimulating training areas such as geriatrics [12,13]. One humorous but biting evaluation of the problems with medical school curricula in particular labeled them "diseases of the curriculum" [14]. These included *curriculosclerosis* or "hardening of the categories," an extreme case of departmentalization; *curriculoarthritis,* a condition limiting articulation between adjacent elements of the curriculum; *curriculum hypertrophy,* or the adding of new knowledge without removing any outdated information. Of particular relevance here is *intercurrent curriculitis,* which describes the inability of the curriculum to be responsive to current societal needs and priorities, for example, the care of the elderly.

Some Hopeful Prospects

Despite this rather gloomy picture, there are some hopeful portents that the situation for interdisciplinary training and practice in geriatrics is improving and will continue to do so. First, there is evidence of increased interest and concern about the problem by groups of physicians, not only those in the vanguard, such as members of the American Geriatrics Society, but others as well. One report cited the need for physicians to be more aware of the skills of allied health professionals and to make more use of existing community-based services in order to provide more comprehensive care for their patients [15]. Perhaps some of this interest by physicians is generated by elderly patients who are showing signs of expecting more holistic treatment from their physicians. Although at present elderly patients are less likely than middle-aged ones to challenge the physician's authority or to make special demands, it is predicted that the next generation of elderly will be more knowledgeable about their condition and more demanding about participating in decision-making with their doctors [16].

A second promising trend is that attitudes of medical students toward the elderly can become more positive if the right kind of training experiences are made available [17] and, I would add, if the right kind of role models can be employed. To be sure, not all reports of student attitudes show a favorable change because of the sensitivity of expressed attitudes to situational characteristics. Nonetheless, there is considerable evidence about the effects of appropriate role models and challenging learning situations [18,19]. A recent issue of the *Journal of the American Geriatrics Society* contained several articles implicitly acknowledging these factors in the recommendations for training at both the undergraduate and graduate levels as well as for continuing education [20].

Third, efforts to establish interdisciplinary training programs in geriatrics are springing up in a variety of settings, including university-based medical centers, community hospitals, and special programs in family medicine. A recent conference on geriatric education, sponsored by the American Association of Retired People (AARP), brought together several hundred representatives from programs that varied widely in the degree of development, the organizational base, the target population, and the amount of available resources. Nonetheless, the extent of expressed interest and commitment to geriatrics was encouraging. In addition, there are reports of new programs that make use of community settings to introduce students to the well elderly as well as to sensitize students to the special needs of the sick elderly [21]. Others emphasize the importance of good preceptors, especially in settings other than acute hospitals [22]. Furthermore, postgraduate fellowship programs have been established in interdisciplinary centers, such as those offered at the geriatric research, evaluation and clinical care centers in Veterans Administration Hospitals.

I believe there is more interest in and greater resources for interdisciplinary training in geriatrics than one might suspect. At least this is true of the experience at St. Louis University. In the process of responding to a federal initiative for support for geriatric training, we found many people already involved in relevant training or in practice and many more who only needed the opportunity to become active. We began modestly enough by identifying individuals in the medical school—especially in the departments of internal medicine, psychiatry, neurology, and community medicine. Several individuals in these departments were conducting geriatric training and research more or less independently and worked with those few students who showed an interest. Simply making these individuals aware of each other's efforts has stimulated exploration of ways to collaborate. Others in the medical school faculty, including basic science departments, were identified as well.

More important to the goal of interprofessional training, individuals in other units of the medical center and the larger university faculty were identified and added to the roster of resource personnel. These included professionals already committed to geriatrics in nursing, the physician assistant program, physical therapy, hospital administration, social work, and the graduate program operated by the university's Institute for Applied Gerontology. Finally, we added to our resource panel persons from local community agencies that serve the elderly, for example, area agencies on aging, home health agencies, public health departments, and the private practice of medicine. We are now working to coordinate the skills of these personnel and the resources we have identified to provide an extensive as well as intensive learning milieu in geriatrics for students in the health professions as well as in continuing education for established practitioners.

The fourth trend is policy statements that favor training and practice in geriatrics. For example, in 1977, members of the American Geriatrics Society made some recommendations regarding geriatric education that included [20]:

1. Further integrating geriatrics into existing training programs, especially in undergraduate medical education.
2. Stimulating an interest in aging in faculty in several disciplines.

3. Establishing interdisciplinary centers on aging to bring together those with interest and experience in geriatrics and long-term care.
4. Using varied settings in ambulatory care to emphasize prevention and re-habilitation and long-term-care alternatives, such as day care and home care.

These policy recommendations clearly call for increased collaboration among health professional groups.

More recently a policy statement and specific recommendations were issued by the Institute of Medicine of the National Academy of Sciences [23]. This report surveyed the current status of training in gerontology and geriatrics in medical education, identified some key elements in the knowledge base, and recommended that resident training should occur in multidisciplinary settings with adequate staffing in nursing, social work, and applied health professionals.

References

1. Siegel, J.S. Prospective trends in the size and structure of the elderly population. *Current Popul. Rep. Spec. Studies.* Series P-23. No. 78. January, 1979.

2. Albrecht, G.L. (Ed.) *Sociology of Physical Disability and Rehabilitation.* Pittsburgh: University of Pittsburgh Press, 1976.

3. Cottrell, L. and Sheldon, E. Problems of collaboration between social scientists and the practicing professions. *Ann. Amer. Acad. Pol. Soc. Sci.* 346: 126, 1963.

4. Freidson, E. *Professional Dominance.* New York: Atherton, 1970.

5. Zola, I.K. In the name of health and illness: On some socio-political consequences of medical influence. *Soc. Sci. Med.* 9:83, 1975.

6. Freidson, E. *Profession of Medicine.* New York: Dodd Mead, 1970.

7. Gruber, H.W. Physician attitudes and medical school training. *J. Amer. Ger. Soc.* 25:494, 1977.

8. Akpom, C.A. and Mayer, S. A survey of geriatric education in U.S. medical schools. *J. Med. Educ.* 53:66, 1978.

9. Holtzman, J.M., Toewe, C.H., and Beck, J.D. Specialty preference and attitudes toward the aged, *J. Fam. Prac.* 9:667, 1979.

10. West, J.P. and Stevens, M.D. Comparative analysis of community health planning: Transition from CHA to HSAs. *J. Hlth. Pol. Policy. Law.* 1:193, 1976.

11. Margolis, E. Changing disease patterns, changing values, problems of geriatric care in the U.S.A.: An outsiders view. *Med. Care.* 17:1119, 1979.

12. Anderson, P.C. Obstacles to change in medical education. *J. Med. Educ.* 45:139, 1970.

13. Kutner, M.G. Medical students' orientation toward the chronically ill. *J. Med. Educ.* 53:111, 1978.

14. Abrahamson, S. Disease of the curriculum. *J. Med. Educ.* 53:951, 1978.

15. Kassel, V. Geriatrics practice: Moving it from the back burner. *Geriat.* 34:95, 1979.

16. Haug, M. The doctor-patient relationship and the old patient. *J. Geront.* 34:852, 1979.

17. Holtzman, J.M., Beck, J.D., and Coggan, P.G. Geriatrics program for medical students. II. Impact of the educational experiences on student attitudes. *J. Amer. Geriat. Soc.* 26:355, 1978.

18. Merton, R.K., Reader, G.G., and Kendell, P. *The Student-Physician.* Cambridge, Mass.: Harvard University Press, 1957.

19. Becker, H.S., Geer, B., Hughes, E.C., and Strauss, A. *Boys in White.* Chicago: University of Chicago Press, 1961.

20. Reichel, W. (Ed.). Proceedings of the American Geriatrics Society Conferences on Geriatric Education. *J. Amer. Ger. Soc.* 25:485, 1977.

21. Birenbaum, A., Aronson, M., and Seiffer, S. Training Medical Students to Appreciate the Special Problems of the Elderly. *Geront.* 19:575, 1979.

22. Williams, T.F., Izzo, A.J., and Steel, R.K. Innovations in teaching about chronic illness and aging in a chronic disease hospital. In D.W. Clark and T.F. Williams (Eds.). *Teaching about Chronic Illness and Aging.* Washington, D.C., DHEW Pub #(NIH) 75-876, Bethesda, MD, 1973.

23. Institute of Medicine. *Aging and Medical Education.* Washington, D.C.: National Academy of Sciences, 1978.

31

The School of Social Work-School of Medicine Connection

Bess Dana, M.S.S.A.

The current efforts of medical education to atone for its long neglect of the health needs and problems of the aging and the aged appear to represent a natural opportunity to bring schools of medicine and schools of social work together in common cause. Indeed, there is knowledge to be shared and guilt to be acknowledged, for neither profession knows enough to deal alone with the wonders and complexities of aging as a bio-psycho-social process. What Elaine Brody (personal communication) defines as a full "moral as well as intellectual commitment" to the enhancement of the social health care of the elderly carries with it the need for medicine and social work to resolve the differences that have characterized their relationship and to find creative ways of using interprofessional educational means to achieve effective interprofessional ends.

An essential first step in the activation of interprofessionalism in the practice of geriatric medicine and social work is to rescue the term "interprofessionalism" from the sea of semantic confusion in which it is currently immersed and to try to bring conceptual order to bear on curriculum development and implementation. Is interprofessionalism, as common usage would suggest, synonymous with teamwork? Can the word "interdisciplinary" be substituted, as it so frequently is, for the word "interprofessional" without altering, albeit subtly, the true meaning of each term? Does interprofessionalism in fact stand for a set of distinguishing behavioral characteristics from which specific educational objectives can be derived?

The views on the relationship between medical and social work education that follow are based on the assumption that the concept of interprofessionalism has its own integrity. It derives its unique character from the bonding of the substances of the various biological, social, and behavioral science disciplines with the various stylistic expressions of collaboration, such as teamwork and consultation. To meet this definition, interprofessional education for medicine and social work must be based on an interdisciplinary frame of reference for viewing health and disease. Opportunities must be provided for social work and medical students to bring their different perspectives to bear in the application of this frame of reference to the identification and solution of the health problems of individuals, groups, and communities. Implied in this interpretation of

The author wishes to express particular thanks to Elaine and Stanley Brody for their generous sharing of their writings and ideas.

193

the requirements of interprofessional education are the encouragement of the capacity to accept and work with difference and the willingness on the part of each profession to give up its insistence on autonomy and substitute interdependence as an essential condition of professionalism.

The ability to satisfy these expectations for interprofessional education is in large measure determined by the knowledge, skills, and attitudes honored and set in motion through professional education. Criteria for the selection of students, the range of professions and disciplines represented in the faculty, the crossing of departmental lines in the governance of the professional school, the role of faculty in university and community affairs, the stance toward learning and teaching conveyed through faculty-student interactions in formal and informal learning experiences—all these conditions of professional education must be recognized along with the content and organization of the formal curriculum itself as the forces that promote or retard interprofessional learning and doing.

Ideally, criteria for admission to schools of medicine and schools of social work should reflect a recognition of the importance of the applicant's potential for interprofessional engagement by noting the breadth as well as the depth of the applicant's academic program and extracurricular activities. Efforts should be made to reward evidence of the capacity to work with others as well as scholastic achievement, paying serious attention to the applicant's social concerns and the avenues through which they have been expressed.

Likewise, the selection and deployment of faculty should, in the best of all interprofessional worlds, reflect not only an appropriate balance among the various professions and disciplines needed to implement a bio-psycho-social frame of reference as essential to medicine and social work education but give special recognition, in appointments and promotions, to a demonstrated capacity to accept both the strengths and limitations of each area of expertise and to learn from as well as teach with others, including students. Finally, if the spirit of interprofessionalism is to permeate the fabric of professional education, full advantage should be taken of the theoretical opportunity that university membership provides for the exchange of ideas among departments and schools in the determination of school and university policy, for the crossing of departmental and school lines in the accomplishment of agreed-upon educational goals, and for the strengthening of the university's role as an instrument of the larger society.

Few of these conditions for setting the spirit, art, and acts of interprofessionalism in motion prevail in the present climate of either medical or social work education. Instead, in their formative professional years, both medical and social work students are exposed to the obstacles that each professional school encounters in keeping *intra*professionalism as the conditioning process for *inter*professionalism alive and well. A number of factors encourage the status quo: the uncontrolled growth of specialized knowledge, the competing demands of both science and society, and the fickle nature of governmental support on which both medical and social work education increasingly rely for survival.

Medical students thus find the road toward professional identity as a physician marked by a series of seemingly disconnected curricular paths, detours, and road blocks. They speak to the lack of unity between the so-called basic and clinical sciences of medicine, the continuing uneasiness about permitting the social and behavioral sciences to enter the mainstream of preparation for careers in medicine, and the barriers created against enlarging curricular space to accommodate community-side as well as bedside teaching and learning.

It takes a highly motivated, resourceful student to find a professional sense of self as a future doctor whose understanding of the role and responsibilities of doctoring transcends the various areas of specialization to include, for all physicians:

1. An acceptance of self as a central but not an exclusive figure in health and medical care.
2. An appreciation of the fact that the physician's responsibilities, like those of the other members of the health and medical care system are influenced not only by the standards of his profession but by the needs, goals and resources of the patient, family and community.
3. The ability to render health services in a way that reflects an understanding of the interplay between biomedical and psychosocial circumstances in influencing the capacity to achieve optimal social health functioning.
4. The capacity to work with other professional and nonprofessional colleagues, patients, and families in the interest of the patient.
5. The concomitant capacity to give way to others whose services can be more relevant than physicians' services at a particular moment in time and at the same time maintain interests in and concern about the patient.[1]

Social work students, no less than medical students, often find the very process of becoming a social worker tends to obscure as much as to clarify the quintessential meaning of being a social worker. Like the medical student, the social work student is subjected to an educational program that reflects persistent difficulties in defining the generic knowledge base for the profession, in establishing and maintaining viable linkages among the various specialties through which the elusive common base is theoretically expected to be expressed, and in easing the chronic tensions between town and gown. These identity problems of social work education are compounded by what appears to be increasing uncertainty as to social work's central purpose, expressed educationally as a growing rift between those who would educate for social change and those who would educate for individual change.

In common with the medical student, the social work student too must be self-reliant and resourceful in the attainment of those attributes of the professional self that promote and facilitate the capacity to work with and through others in identifying and solving social health problems. Required are:

1. A sense of professional self-worth, based on an acceptance of what social work stands for and a beginning grasp of the knowledge and skills through which this stance is expressed.
2. A concomitant acceptance of the limitations of social work knowledge and skills in the face of the multifaceted nature and manifestations of social health problems.
3. The capacity for lateral thinking articulated through the establishment, maintenance, and promotion of linkages, such as those between the individual and society, the consumer and the provider, prevention and treatment, and so on.
4. The willingness to put social needs and goals, whether individually, institutionally, or universally expressed, ahead of professional self-interests in the definition and implementation of social work tasks and responsibilities.

The role model that the enterprising or just plain lucky medical or social work student happens to encounter in the search for ways to support and sustain a wavering belief in holism; the serendipitous learning derived from the patient whose social and psychological needs defy the biomedical message he or she is supposed to convey; the chance meeting between social work and medical student in the course of their pursuits of independent learning assignments; the planned elective that brings medical and social work students together one afternoon a week for six or eight weeks to study family dynamics, human sexuality, health policy; the participation of social workers in medical school instruction in interviewing, in clinical correlations, in teaching rounds; the participation of psychiatrists, pediatricians, even, occasionally, internists in the human growth and behavior sequences in schools of social work; the "umbrella" course offered on a few campuses as a learning requirement for all students in the health professions—this mixture of planned and accidental educational opportunities represents the resources on which, with few exceptions, America's medical and social work students rely in order to satisfy the behavioral prerequisites for the seeding of interprofessionalism. At their best, these kinds of learning experiences can serve to sustain and inspire the student's sense of social purpose, expand his or her professional horizons, substitute the satisfactions of collaboration for the tensions of competition, and begin to provide the glimmerings of the role and responsibilities of other health professions and disciplines in health and medical care.

These positive outcomes are, however, by no means universal. Because of the elective nature of most of the learning experiences that promote the development of interprofessionalism, they are likely to have their most favorable impact on self-propelling students whose sense of professional direction is strong enough to permit them to grasp each educational opportunity. The large proportion of today's student body is less likely to wander away from the prescribed educational program, even in the selection of electives in order to explore alternative routes toward professionalism. All students have the right to expect that the required curriculum, rather than elective study or chance learning, will expose them to the essential intellectual, attitudinal, and skill components of their chosen profession. To bring about a reversal of the usual ways in which students are prepared for their interdependent futures, however, necessitates educational action that goes beyond the constant reiteration of the theoretical rationale for interprofessional education; the gloomy assessment of the prospects for converting theory into practice; or the simplistic solutions to complex problems that so much of the professional literature reflects. Instead, medical and social work educators who wish to bring about change might direct their energies toward:

1. A critical examination of their respective educational behaviors as they promote or impede the climate as well as the content of intraprofessional and interprofessional learning.
2. Formal and informal assessment of the strengths and limitations of the intraprofessional and interprofessional components of their respective educational programs from the perspective of the students, faculty, and representatives of the health and medical care practice community.
3. Joint exploration of the knowledge and attitudes that social workers and physicians hold with respect to each other's professional goals and objectives, the characteristics of the educational programs through which the knowledge, values, and skills of each professional are transmitted, and the educational issues at the forefront of concern.
4. The formation and maintenance of a continuing curriculum development group charged with responsibility for the determination of mutual learning needs, the translation of learning needs into educational objectives, and the design, implementation, and evaluation of specific learning experiences (didactic and experiential) through which educational objectives become curriculum realities.

This developmental approach to interprofessional education places a strong emphasis on process as a powerful determinant of outcome.

    The ordering and tasks of the developmental phases that have been described represent an attempt to convert into an interrelated series of anticipatory educational activities the remedial measures that many of us have resorted to in our efforts to save or maintain interprofessional relationships in our lives as practitioners or teachers. For example, who among us, whose interprofessional design has survived beyond the initial period of outside funding to achieve institutional support and status has not learned that there are no shortcuts to either intraprofessional or interprofessional accord—that conflict cannot be avoided but must be faced? Who, once the first shock of the students' solicited or gratuitous affront to our educational sense and sensibilities has abated, has not found it productive to make our seemingly most merciless student critic as well as our most ardent student supporter a participant in the solution rather than a perpetrator of the problem? Who has not discovered, too often only after the resources of the academic environment have proved insufficient to the task, the rich educational yield to be derived from those who *do* interprofessionalism?

The tradition of separatism within and between schools of social work and schools of medicine is too firmly embedded, to establish "instant" interprofessionalism in the field of geriatrics. However, it appears to be possible to make educational attention to aging the basis for a revitalization of interprofessionalism that will enhance the capacity of medicine and social work to serve people of all ages.

If the lessons of the past as interpreted in this chapter are to be incorporated as guidelines for the initiation and implementation of this revitalization process, then the process itself will reflect:

The importance of making geriatric education an integral component of the total preparation of all students in both medicine and social work.

The activation of this charge to medical and social work education as a whole through 1) participation of faculty representatives from both schools in the tasks of self-assessment designed as the first phase of the developmental process as well as in the other phases of curriculum development, implementation, and evaluation process, and 2) the extension of the scope of inquiry beyond the formal curriculum to encompass an assessment of what is "caught" as well as taught.

The recognition that the design and implementation of interprofessional learning experiences are not likely to evolve successfully without meeting and dealing with conflicting values, correcting for lack of knowledge of each other's programs, and sacrificing the security afforded by autonomy.

The concomitant acceptance of faculty development as an integral component of curriculum development for interprofessional engagement, with all that implies by way of openness to learning from students, from practitioners, as well as from faculty colleagues.

The articulation of the principles of interprofessional behavior in the style as well as substance of interprofessional learning and teaching through such measures as 1) the participation of faculty from other professions and disciplines in medical and social work education, 2) the provision of conjoint learning opportunities of both a didactic and experiential nature, and 3) the involvement of practitioners and consumers of services in classroom and experiential learning.

The expansion of the learning space to include conjoint experiential learning opportunities outside the hospital—in the home, the long-term facility, and the community center.

The acknowledgment of the primacy of the aging person and family.

In summary then, education for interprofessional education, whether directed toward understanding and meeting the social health needs of the aging and aged or toward serving the general population, is essentially education in interrelationships. The aging as a population group epitomize the interdependence of all these factors as they interact to determine the nature and form of the human condition. If we can begin to act on the concept of the aging as the teachers of all of us, then the elderly can once again assume their traditional role in influencing the quality and expression of the medical-social work relationship in all areas of human service.

Note

1. Adapted from Bess Dana, "A Proposed Learning-Teaching Model for Undergraduate Medical Education in Comprehensive Patient Health Care Management," *Milbank Memorial Fund* Quarterly, Volume XLVII, October 1969.

32

The Geriatric AHEC at the University of Maryland: A Model for Geriatric Education

Morton Rapoport, M.D.
Barbara Cahn, M.S.W.

The Geriatric Area Health Education Center (AHEC) at the University of Maryland at Baltimore began in October 1979. This interdisciplinary education/service program was developed for students from the University's six professional schools: Dentistry, Law, Medicine, Nursing, Pharmacy, and Social Work and Community Planning, as well as for the general community. Since the primary thrust of the AHEC initiative is remote or community-based education, sites include clinics for the elderly in highrise apartments, a large multipurpose senior center, a community hospital outpatient department, and a Veterans Administration Hospital Primary Care Clinic. Several established community facilities for the elderly were designated Geriatric AHEC sites. In these sites, multidisciplinary teams of faculty and students provide primary-care services to the aged within a structured educational environment. This chapter describes the interaction between national initiatives and priorities in aging, existing strengths, and established programs at the University of Maryland at Baltimore, and how they were blended into the unique outreach thrust called the Geriatric AHEC.

In 1970 the Carnegie Commission published a report on higher education and the nation's health. This study highlighted the national problem of maldistribution of medical resources. According to the report, services were concentrated in middle-class urban areas, with few resources for poor or rural populations. In addition, the number of primary-care clinicians was declining as the trend toward specialization increased. The Commission proposed decentralized health-manpower-education programs under supervision of academic health centers. As a result of this report, the first Area Health Education Bill was passed by Congress in 1972, and money was appropriated to the Health Resources Administration to promote innovative health education programs.

The professional schools of the University of Maryland responded to this federal initiative in 1976 by developing an AHEC in Western Maryland, in the Allegheny-Garrett County Appalachian region. Students from the Schools of Medicine, Dentistry, Social Work and Community Planning, Nursing (Nurse Practitioners), and Pharmacy fulfilled part of their clinical training requirements in this nonurban area. Students were assigned to selected clinicians in western Maryland who served as preceptors.

As a result of the favorable experience with the western Maryland AHEC and in response to increasing interest by the six professional schools in aging, the University of Maryland proposed a population-based AHEC as a supplement to the geographic AHEC program. It is widely recognized that health-care providers and institutions have been insensitive and unresponsive to the needs of the aged. It was reasoned that maldistribution of health professionals occurred not only on a regional and specialty basis but also on a population basis.

Income maintenance and health and social programs for the elderly are being developed nationwide. However, geriatric education has lagged behind the implementation of concrete services. Existing programs for the elderly embody a categorical approach and are based on an ideology that emphasizes the unique characteristics of the aged. This specialized focus has been translated by educational institutions into programs and centers on aging and departments of geriatrics. Developments at the University of Maryland at Baltimore have followed this categorical trend.

In 1978 the Task Force on Aging was created at the University of Maryland at Baltimore (UMAB) to coordinate and stimulate geriatric education in the six professional schools. In an effort to develop a geriatric focus within the university, the task force capitalized on existing strengths, many of which had not been considered geriatric resources. It became a coalition of professional schools' deans as well as leaders of academic geriatrics.

In addition, a number of situational factors at UMAB facilitated acceptance of the Task Force on Aging. At the time of its inception, a Center on Aging had already been in existence for three years at the University of Maryland at College Park—the largest undergraduate and graduate school campus. The center was able to generate seed money to establish the task force, as well as to share specialized knowledge and skills. Although six professional schools exist on one campus in Baltimore, the degree of interprofessionalism had been minimal. However, shortly before the creation of the Task Force on Aging, a Vice-Chancellor's Office for Health Affairs had been created as a focal point for interprofessional activities, and the Dean of the School of Medicine was appointed to be the first Vice-Chancellor. The task force thus became a Vice-Chancellor's program and benefited from a defined role in the University's organizational structure. Also, the success of an interprofessional primary-care initiative and liberal approaches to the development of nonphysician providers had begun to bridge the gaps between professions.

The initial efforts of the task force were directed toward the identification of areas of interest in aging in the six professional schools and the gaining of high visibility for geriatric education. The Colloquium on Aging has featured, on various occasions, Lillian Carter, Arthur Flemming, Robert Benedict, and Robert Butler. The spring colloquium, chaired by a task force member and the wife of the governor, served as a stimulus for gaining student and faculty interest in aging. With maturation of the task force in terms of experience and recognition on the campus, it naturally assumed the responsibility of organization and implementation of the Geriatric AHEC program.

The Task Force on Aging recognized that the Geriatric AHEC concept embodied their belief that community-based programs are essential for geriatric education. It was agreed that student exposure should go beyond the hospital and nursing home and should include familiarization with family and community support systems for the aged. Fortunately, a model for community care already existed at UMAB within the Division of Primary Care of the Department of Medicine and could be modified to include a geriatric focus. This model of professional education and health-care delivery emphasized service integration. Furthermore, the leadership role of the UMAB campus in developing and supporting the concept of nonphysician primary-care providers including nurse practitioners and clinical pharmacists was viewed as a factor favoring the interprofessional initiative in aging education and service delivery. The role of these nonphysician professionals in the education of many types of students for the provision of chronic stable primary care was of considerable assurance to the administrative staff on the Geriatric AHEC in its planning stages.

The Geriatric AHEC provided UMAB with a clinical program in which many of the theoretical constructs developed by the Task Force on Aging and the primary care programs could be employed. Geriatric clinics in community settings were established, and existing clinics were modified to be more in keeping with the goals outlined. Students were exposed both to a cross-section of the elderly population and to the complexities of service delivery. In addition, since the AHEC was a novel program, new models of service delivery and coordination as well as geriatric education could be developed.

Some professionals maintain that fragmentation of service to the elderly occurs as a result of inappropriate emphases on the medical model of human service delivery at the expense of the social model. Furthermore, service providers must understand the roles and objectives of professions other than their own so as to permit care plans to reflect more efficient and less redundant interventions.

UMAB faculty recognized that a major impediment to interprofessionalism was inadequate curriculum development. Consequently, the Task Force on Aging established an education subcommittee to address this problem. The committee, composed of representatives of the six professional schools, first established minimum-practice entry competencies in aging for each of the six professions. This document served as the foundation for discipline-specific curriculum development and highlighted the many common ideal competencies that the professions shared. These common or interprofessional competencies became the basis for common curricular and programmatic development (table 32-1). The ability to conceptualize what each professional requires in basic and spe-

Table 32–1

Basic Minimum Competencies for Professional Students (Medicine, Dentistry, Law, Social Work, Pharmacy, Nursing) in Geriatric Outreach Facilities

Objectives	Cognitive Competencies	Skills	Affective Competencies
Describe and understand the roles of the health-care team.	Explain the structure of the outreach program and the relationship between faculty, health-care team and student.	Be able to work as a professional within the interprofessional structure.	Develop appreciation of how the team structure relates to individual skills of the various team members.
Understand the organizational structure of the geriatric facility.	Understand management techniques, strategy development and organizational planning.	Be able to develop an organizational structure that will facilitate team management.	Understand the relationship of theory to practice in the outreach site.
Function as a member of the interdisciplinary health-care team and as a provider of direct care.	1. Be aware of the mechanics of interdisciplinary health care for the elderly—know the skill, functions and roles of professionals in other disciplines. 2. Know principles of group dynamics.	1. Demonstrate effective communication skills for relating to patients and colleagues. 2. Be able to work effectively within a multidisciplinary team. 3. Be able to formulate an interdisciplinary treatment plan. 4. Be able to perform triage with the geriatric patient. 5. Be able to facilitate group interaction through competent application of the principles of group dynamics.	1. Develop appreciation of and respect for the competencies. 2. Appreciate the necessity and value of interdisciplinary care for the elderly.
Understand the basic principles of geriatrics.	1. Be aware of the local, state, federal and private resources available to the elderly. 2. Develop an awareness of social, economic, psychological and physiological factors which influence the behavior of the elderly. 3. Understand the political and economic environment and its implications for geriatric medicine. 4. Understand the demography and epidemiology of the geriatric population.	Be able to engage community services and to recognize the need for auxiliary supports.	1. Develop positive attitudes toward older people. 2. Develop a sensitivity to the social, economic, physiological and psychological factors which affect the elderly.

204

cialized education enabled the education subcommittee to mold an interprofessional AHEC model. Innovations in intake interviews, case sharing and conferencing, and core conferences evolved from this competency framework.

Although the professional schools at the University of Maryland all had clinical programs, their experience and success with community-based outreach education had differed. Social work has always utilized the field experience, whereas this is not the case for legal education. Dentistry and medicine had been accustomed to education within the environs of their own institutions and only recently have begun to look beyond university-sponsored facilities. However, the fact that a required community clinical experience existed within the curricula of each school was important. The Geriatric AHEC was able to include students assigned to community rotations and thus did not have to significantly change existing academic programs and schedules. The schools were receptive to a geriatric interprofessional community experience and willingly developed AHEC placements. In fact, some of the schools saw the AHEC as the vehicle for expanding community clinical education.

There were very important practical issues in program implementation:

1. *Coordination of Six Disciplines.* As stated previously, there are great variations in the need for and structure of clinical rotations at the six professional schools. For example, the School of Social Work and Community Planning assigns students to one agency placement for 30 hours per week for 9 months during both years of a two-year master's degree program. The law and nursing schools assign students to clinical placements a few hours a week for a full semester. The dental and pharmacy schools have four-week full-time senior rotations with community providers, and the School of Medicine has four-day-per-week eight-week ambulatory care rotations in medical clinics for fourth-year students. Developing a schedule in which all schools can participate in clinical as well as didactic experiences has required extensive negotiation. At each site, one day has been designated "interprofessional" and all schools participate in case and core conferences as well as service delivery. Core sessions are designed on an eight-week schedule. Since some students spend more than eight weeks in a setting, they are utilized as "facilitators" for group presentations. Each school assigns a faculty preceptor to each AHEC site. The schools of medicine, pharmacy and dentistry require that preceptors must be present during student clinical encounters. For the remaining schools, faculty supervise students but do not participate in the direct clinical process. Student/faculty clinical services and educational programs at each site are coordinated by the AHEC Director and an on-site nurse practitioner.

2. *Implementation of the Curriculum.* The Geriatric AHEC curriculum was based on the minimum competencies developed by the education subcommittee of the Task Force on Aging. This curriculum concentrates on areas of importance to each discipline as well as the interprofessional competencies that all

professionals should master. Implementation of the curriculum has required a great deal of flexibility by the six professional schools. It involved modification of existing one-to-one practices as well as adaptation of nontraditional techniques. In order to refine the model, the curriculum was tested in a primary-care clinic during the fall semester. Preceptors met weekly to discuss issues of integration and coordination. The group process helped to modify the program and to insure its applicability to the educational mission of the AHEC. By including preceptors in the endeavor, their investment and understanding of the program has increased.

3. *Relationship with the Baltimore Community.* In order to develop a viable AHEC program, it was essential to involve the organized Baltimore community in this process. Education through community outreach is a relatively new concept in geriatric education. However, a wealth of programs for the elderly exist in the Baltimore area, which are invaluable resources for the AHEC. A broad-based advisory committee was developed that included policy-makers, representatives of state and local government, service providers, retired professionals as well as persons from the academic community. Initial meetings of the advisory committee were devoted to a thorough explanation of the educational mission. Issues, such as the impact of students on existing patterns of service delivery and the potential benefits to the general population, were explored. The community representatives may have had initial reservations regarding an interface with the university in their sphere but were overwhelmingly supportive of a program for educating tomorrow's professional and potentially enhancing service to the elderly. Some persons in the university were skeptical about the community's participation in an education program. However, an active executive committee composed of the director of the state office on aging, the mayor's coordinator of human resources, the director of a large multipurpose senior center as well as high-level representatives from the schools of medicine, dentistry, and social work, and staff familiar with both the academic and service communities, helped to minimize tension between the community and the university.

4. *Issues of Site Selection.* A site subcommittee of the advisory committee developed a list of criteria for site selection. Existing clinical settings were sought which could serve an elderly population, accommodate a variety of professional students and faculty, and institute an interprofessional model. A major issue was continuity. Providers feared service would suffer as patients were seen by a variety of students. In order to minimize lack of continuity, sites were selected in which education would overlay existing services that continued regardless of student availability. The AHEC did not want to establish new settings but to utilize community resources and hopefully to enhance care through its educational innovations. Fortunately, the advisory committee's acceptance of the AHEC concept helped the program to gain access to a variety of outstanding facilities. Rather than considering the program as interfering with service de-

livery, the community perceived AHEC as complementing it. Requests for participation in the program outnumber present faculty/student capacity. Final site selection reflected the committee's and the staff's desire to expose students to a diverse elderly population, who utilize a variety of community resources.

5. *Evaluation.* Evaluation instruments have been developed that assess student and faculty attitudes toward this program. Scales have been developed to explore knowledge and attitudes toward the elderly as well as toward the inter-. professional model. It is too early to assess the impact of this program. The first groups of students and preceptors expressed increased awareness of other professions as well as heightened sensitivity toward and acceptance of the elderly population.

The University of Maryland at Baltimore made a conscious decision to approach the teaching of geriatrics from a community perspective in order to generate a realistic understanding of the aging process. The Geriatric AHEC helped to create interest and enthusiasm regarding aging among students and faculty and to facilitate interschool cooperation. Furthermore, both the University and the community at large have begun to recognize mutual dependencies as well as potential benefits to both education and service.

By allowing for a broad-based input in program design and implementation, there has been considerable investment in this project by all of the schools involved. It is hoped that recognition of the potential of this novel program for education and research in problems of the aged will increase and that the success of this initial effort will stimulate other education and research initiatives in geriatrics in each of the six professional schools.

Appendixes

The Geriatric Momentum: So Much Verbiage or Social Progress?

Stanley R. Ingman, Ph.D.

Academic medicine must be careful not to abuse the federal and lay trust. First, if academic centers channel funding into traditional biomedical research programs to the exclusion of geriatric clinical practice and long-term care, they will set geriatrics back ten years.

Second, the aged should also be concerned that neither family medicine nor internal medicine capture the new turf, geriatric medicine. Both have unique contributions to make to the evolving definition of geriatric practice in hospitals, long-term-care facilities, outpatient settings and the home.

Third, a small group of geriatric consultants (specialists) in the United States would not fragment the doctor-patient relationship significantly. Geriatric specialization in Europe has not meant that the elderly have been required to go to a new physician for overall care. Rather, most aged have remained under the care of a general practitioner. (This is especially true in Denmark.)

As discussed by David Carboni, Ph.D., some form of geriatric specialty can help the family practitioner, internist, and subspecialist improve their own care of older individuals. Medical students are increasingly interested in geriatric practice, but it continues to be difficult for academic centers to point to successful practice situations or career opportunities. Without some genuine geriatric faculty and without community geriatric physicians devoting themselves to the organizational as well as the clinical issues, the public will soon question the benefit of the recent surge in federal expenditures in this area.

The Effect of the Site of Clinical Experience on the Attitudes of the Student

L. Gregory Pawlson, M.D.
Valery A. Portnoi, M.D.
Jean E. Johnson, N.P.
Kevin R. Sorem, P.A.-C.

It is apparent that a wide range of sites are currently being used to provide clinical experiences in geriatric medicine. Training programs must often make use first of those sites that are readily available in their particular locale. Further, it has been proposed that learning is dependent more on the enthusiasm of the teacher than on the particular site. Yet, there are few descriptive accounts and fewer studies of the effect of site on attitudes and learning. It is possible that some sites might have a major negative impact on both learning and attitudes. Medical students, medical residents, nurse practitioners, and physicians' assistants at George Washington University are involved in geriatric clinical experiences in a congregate housing project with a senior activity center, a medical center hospital, two long-term-care facilities (one nonprofit, one government) and an outpatient geriatric evaluation unit. We postulate that the specific site and sequence of experiences has an important effect on changes in attitude toward the elderly as well as retention of specific knowledge. We have formulated a number of hypotheses, such as 1) early exposure to the congregate housing population in an interviewing course enables the student to recognize that the majority of elderly persons are capable of self care and are mentally sound and 2) the nursing home experience has a negative impact on attitudes and makes knowledge acquisition difficult unless accompanied by some discussion of the feelings that the student experiences in this environment. A formal study of the effect of the site and the sequence of training experiences on these and other hypotheses dealing with student attitudes and knowledge has been instituted. We would urge other teaching sites to do similar studies, many of which can be done on a very limited research budget in the hope that the information will result in the more appropriate use of sites and insure the best possible geriatric education for health science students.

Categorical versus Noncategorical Units for the Teaching of Geriatrics

Carol Winograd, M.D.

Delivery of health-care services to geriatric patients can be approached from two different perspectives: categorical (age-segregated) or noncategorical (non-age-segregated). There are pros and cons of both.

In a categorical geriatric ward or clinic, the staff can be taught principles of geriatric care, and a team approach can be mobilized with the pace and organization of care geared to the needs of the older patient. Furthermore, patient care and teaching can be focused in one setting. Students and postgraduate health professionals have ready access to clinical experiences. Moreover, such a geriatric unit can serve as a center for basic science and clinical research. One disadvantage is that both the individuals who staff these units and the principle of a comprehensive team approach utilized in these units can have little impact on the type of care given geriatric patients in other units, due to the physical and psychological separation of the geriatrics unit. The second disadvantage is that such a unit is costly in terms of staff time. It requires a large number of personnel to provide the type of care such geriatric patients require.

Because the goal of both teaching and patient-care programs is to improve the quality of care for all older patients, a noncategorical approach that incorporates geriatric principles in a variety of outpatient and inpatient settings might be more effective. Formal geriatrics teaching rounds on specific cases can provide a spillover of geriatric principles to other patients. Moreover, an interdisciplinary approach to comprehensive care for some patients is likely to lead to similar approaches for all patients.

The disadvantages of a noncategorical approach is that it requires working with a larger number of physicians and other health professionals; it may be harder to develop a sense of team effort among the staff; and the pace and approach to care on many units is geared toward younger patients with acute problems. However, in the long run, these disadvantages can be offset by the clear· advantage of integrating geriatric teaching, patient care, and research into mainstream "first class" medicine.

The Use of an Acute Geriatric Assessment Unit for Undergraduate Education in Geriatric Medicine—The Experience at the University of Saskatchewan

Duncan Robertson, M.D.

Undergraduate medical education in geriatric medicine at the University of Saskatchewan utilizes an acute geriatric assessment unit in a 552-bed university hospital. Following didactic teaching in gerontology and geriatric medicine in the first three years of a five-year medical program, all medical students are attached for one week to the geriatric assessment unit, where they participate as members of the health team.

Students attend in groups of two. The intensive programs include the following:

1. Participation in three case conferences: admission assessment case conference, at which the student presents his patient; discharge planning conference, held weekly for all patients; and day hospital case conference.

2. Participation in daily ward teaching on the management of acute illness in old age and methods of assessing the determinants of breakdown and management of breakdown in independent living in old age.

3. Visits to the homes of patients newly referred to the unit or to patients recently discharged from the acute assessment unit are arranged for each student each week.

4. Participation in the assessment function and other programs of the day hospital.

5. The complete assessment (medical, psychological, functional, social) of an older person admitted to the acute assessment unit.

Students are evaluated on their patient assessment and upon their ability to function in the team setting and communicate with patients, families, and members of the geriatric medicine health team.

Following this mandatory rotation, a number of students return for electives in the fourth medical year, during which a greater degree of responsibility is given to the students.

Use of a Department of Rehabilitation Medicine for the Teaching of Geriatrics

Franz U. Steinberg, M.D.

Consideration of other sites for training is warranted. The Department of Rehabilitation Medicine at the Jewish Hospital of St. Louis/Washington University Medical Center operates a 55-bed service of which a separate 20-bed unit has been set aside for geriatric rehabilitation. Referred from the medical or surgical services of Jewish Hospital and from other hospitals in the metropolitan area, the patients are screened before admission to determine their suitability for a rehabilitation program. Most patients are disabled following a stroke or other neurologic or musculoskeletal disorders, or they suffer from a significant disability following a serious medical illness or surgical operation. General medical care is provided by the patient's private physician if he is a member of the Jewish Hospital staff. This arrangement provides for a better continuity of care. As an additional benefit, this system helps to acquaint the medical staff with the methods and the value of geriatric rehabilitation.

Both the director and the associate director of the service, who are internists as well as psychiatrists, are available for official consultations. The nurses are trained in both rehabilitation and geriatric nursing, which includes an emphasis on training the patients in self-care, restoration of bladder and bowel continence, and ambulation. All services are coordinated in a weekly staff conference, which is attended by the director and the associate director of the service, the head nurse, representative supervisors of the various therapy departments, and the social worker. Approximately 70% of all patients are discharged to their own homes. In many cases, Jewish Hospital's Home Care Program aids in the postdischarge adjustment that patient and family must make.

In addition to residents in physical medicine and rehabilitation and students who are taking rehabilitation as an elective, residents from the Department of Medicine frequently follow patients after their transfer to the Rehabilitation Department. Utilization of traditional rehabilitation programs in the developing geriatric programs should be investigated.

6 Challenges for a Geriatric Consultation Service in the Acute Hospital

Edward W. Campion, M.D.

An inpatient consultative service offers numerous advantages for geriatrics in the acute hospital. It can quickly attain visibility in the midst of a teaching and training environment. It reaches many physicians and patients, maximizing exposure for a small department. A consulting service entails few start-up expenses and no costly political struggles for hospital beds. Indeed, a geriatrician may be surprised to discover strong support from many people already fully aware of the problems of the elderly. Those in social service, psychiatry, nursing, rehabilitation, physical and occupational therapy, recreational therapy, speech therapy, nutrition, chaplaincy, and perhaps even a few physician iconoclasts can be enthusiastic backers. A consulting geriatric team should draw strongly upon these resources. Specific indications for the consultation can be varied: confusion, "failure to thrive," coordination of a rehabilitation program, assessment for placement, or implementation of a difficult discharge to home. A clear definition of the consulting geriatrician's role must be established and communicated.

The role of a consultant specialist is a well-established one familiar to virtually everyone. It implicitly carries respect. Establishing a consultation service broadcasts that the geriatrician represents a body of specialty knowledge just as other valued consultant specialists do. This level of expectation does put the geriatrician under considerable pressure to deliver and to live up to the demands of that role. The opportunities are nearly unlimited for teaching the many unappreciated aspects of geriatric assessment and care.

A new consultation service should be wary of a host of potential problems. If seen simply as a placement service, calls will be numerous and the demand always the same: "Take this patient off my hands." Furthermore, one must be reasonably discreet in making recommendations and not be overly sensitive if some are not accepted. On some crucial issues the geriatrician must be prepared to stand firmly as patient advocate though it can jeopardize popularity. Some physicians may vent upon the geriatrician the anger and frustration they feel for chronically ill elderly persons. Recognizing the wrath of ageism and skillfully seeking its roots can be the greatest challenge of all for a consultant geriatrician.

7

The Geriatric Nurse Practitioner's Role in the Long-Term-Care Setting and its Importance to a Teaching Program—A Personal Experience

John Murphy, R.N.,

When I began my career in nursing in 1937, geriatric nursing and medicine were unknown specialties. A diploma preparation was the usual level of nurse education with B.S. and master's level degrees attained via evening, summer, and sabbatical-leave study. At that ancient date it was frowned upon for a nurse even to take blood pressure.

When the nurse practitioner and physician's assistant programs blossomed in the early 1970s, I was fortunate enough to be accepted into one of the classes at the University of Rochester. My base of experience was in geriatric and long-term-care nursing at Monroe Community Hospital in Rochester, New York, and in the Veteran's Administration Hospital system in New York and California. The course contained material easily applied to the geriatric setting of Monroe Community Hospital where I had spent five years as the Assistant Director of Nursing involved in clinical considerations rather than nursing administration.

In 1973, there were many nurse practitioners in pediatrics, public health, and acute medical and surgical settings. Clinical practice was also common. however, there were no nurse practitioners in long-term-care institutions.

To remedy this, a program was developed in conjunction with the University of Rochester School of Nursing to train nurses specifically for the role of geriatric nurse practitioners in a long-term setting. This effort was superseded at the University of Rochester School of Nursing by incorporating the assessment skills of physical assessment and other pertinent material into the basic degree programs.

Presently, my practice takes place in the large chronic disease facility, the Monroe Community Hospital (MCH), affiliated with the University of Rochester Medical and Dental School. It is staffed entirely by physicians on the staff of the university but is administered by the County of Monroe, which employs most other disciplines including nursing.

I am involved closely with 60 to 70 patients with whom I am in daily contact at three levels of care. Most of them are at the skilled nursing facility (SNF) level of care although a lesser number are at the health related facility (HRF) level of care. A few patients are followed in the clinic or by home visits when it is necessary. These patients are managed with four physicians in eleven separate areas or ward units, the largest of which is a 30-bed unit where I am assigned all of the patients with three of the four physicians. Each physician acts as an attending for his own patients only. It is not a group-type practice.

It is usual to move patients from one level of care to another while continuing the same physician and nurse practitioner coverage. When acute care is needed, the patient is "discharged" to that service but "readmitted" to the same physician and nurse practitioner.

On admission, the nurse practitioner greets the patient, does a history and physical examination, reviews the records available, and prepares a problem list and a proposed plan of medical-nursing care for each problem. If the patient has been on maintenance medications, these are initiated on admission. This work-up is reviewed with the physician within 24 hours, revised as necessary, and implemented by the nurse practitioner. If an acute problem or a life-threatening condition is found, the patient is seen by a physician at once.

Utilization of consulting physicians and services, such as physical therapy, occupational therapy, speech therapy, and podiatry, is implemented by the nurse practitioner as the plan of care is formed. Most nursing-care problems, such as skin care, dressing, and wound care, are managed directly by the nurse practitioner. Family contacts and daily visits are carried out with periodic rounding with a physician for purposes of reviewing the patient's progress and assessing complications. Once the patient has settled into a proscribed therapeutic regimen, the time required of the physician is minimal.

The elements of a successful practice seem to be a mutual confidence between physician and nurse, delegation of responsibility by the physician, adequacy of services within the institution, and 24-hour back-up coverage.

Some of the more technical skills and duties of my practice include: I.V. therapy; gastrostomy, catheter, ileal loop and colostomy management; venous and arterial punctures; management of inhalation therapy (with consultation as need), bowel and bladder management techniques, and incontinence management.

Occasions for teaching are plentiful. The geriatric nurse practitioner is a role model for all nurses in this setting. Most teaching thus takes place at the bedside, where the problems arise.

The University of Rochester School of Nursing, which has baccalaureate to doctoral programs, has utilized this clinical setting to present to their students a complete health-care system for the elderly and chronic long-term-care patient. The experience at MCH permits students to see a patient from the time of admission to the time of placement whether it is back in the home, in another community setting, or as a permanent resident at Monroe Community Hospital. This opportunity is often unavailable to students who otherwise get educated in a classroom or a clinic setting far from the realities of actual practice.

Additionally, it is most important for medical students and house officers to witness how a geriatric nurse practitioner functions in a long-term-care setting. The beneficial effects of the interrelationships of nursing and medicine are being developed in many settings. It is hoped that one of these will be in long-term care.

Issues in Interdisciplinary Geropsychiatric Education

Kenneth Solomon, M.D.

Over 30% of people over the age of 65 will suffer from at least one episode of depression [1] and another 7% will develop one of the dementias [2]. Other psychopathological syndromes, including paraphrenias, personality disorders, anxiety disorders, and adjustment disorders, are also fairly common. Adequate geriatric care requires that health and mental health workers of all professional persuasions be familiar with the basic concepts of recognition, assessment (diagnosis), and intervention (treatment) of older persons with psychiatric difficulties. As these syndromes frequently result from the interaction of multiple biological, psychological, and social factors, it is clear that interdisciplinary work, preferably within a matrix model of team structuring, is absolutely necessary [3].

What is necessary at this time are creative and innovative experiments in the following areas:

1. The development of a basic core interdisciplinary curriculum that would be applicable to primary-care physicians, psychiatrists, nurses, social workers, dentists, attorneys, pharmacists, and clinical psychologists.
2. The development of training packages that allow members of each discipline to be familiar and conversant with the orientation and role behaviors of other disciplines.
3. The formation of a team matrix that allows interdisciplinary role overlap with a maximum of both generalist and specialist role function [3-5] to guarantee access, accountability, and integration of services [3,6-7].
4. The defining of the tasks of a multidisciplinary geropsychiatric team to assure adequate specialty functioning while leaving the responsibility for most geropsychiatric clients with the general clinician. In other words, when is the specialist (geropsychiatrist, gerontologic nurse, and so on) needed?

Although it is clear that the above needs address both educational and service considerations, I believe that they are inseparable. Good clinicians are good teachers and good role models. The need to teach sharpens clinical skills. Until the above issues are addressed, the mental health care of older Americans will remain fragmented and of relatively poor quality.

References

1. Ban, T.A. The treatment of depressed geriatric patients. *Am. J. Psychotherapy* 32:93, 1978.

2. Kay, D.W.K. The epidemiology and identification of brain deficit in the elderly. In C. Eisdorfer and R.O. Friedel (Eds.) *Cognitive and Emotional Disturbance in the Elderly.* Chicago: Year Book Medical Publishers, 1977.

3. Solomon, K. The geropsychiatrist and the delivery of mental health services in the community. Presented at the 32nd Annual Meeting of the Gerontological Society, Washington, D.C. November 26, 1979.

4. Harris, M. and Solomon, K. Roles of the community health nurse. *J. Psychiat. Nurs. Mental Health Services* 15:35, 1977.

5. Solomon, K. The roles of the psychiatric resident on a community psychiatry team. *Psychiat. Quart.,* in press.

6. Gottesman, L.E., Ishizaki, B., and MacBride, S.M. Service management—plan and concept in Pennsylvania. *Gerontologist* 19:379, 1979.

7. Ishizaki, B., Gottesman, L.E., and MacBride, S.M. Determinants of model choice for service management systems. *Gerontologist* 19:385, 1979.

The Psychiatric Home Visit

Jonathan D. Lieff, M.D.

An important principle for geriatric medicine education is that elderly patients can demonstrate psychoneurological symptomatology or somatic medical complaints as a result of emotional, social, or physical problems. Because of this, it is important that psychiatric clinics use new forms of problem-oriented treatment planning that coordinate all aspects of care, including multimodal therapy, psychotherapy, and social work. Proper education, evaluation, and treatment must take all these areas into account.

Second, within this interdisciplinary framework, because of the great impact of environment on the elderly, geriatricians must understand many levels of care, including home care, ambulatory services, nursing homes, as well as inpatient hospital settings. In order to help the elderly maintain independence, aid deinstitutionalization, and best train geriatricians, the unique and important medical tradition of the home visit is invaluable.

There are unique problems in the area of developing a home psychiatric service, not the least of which is that establishing therapeutic bonding for elderly patients takes a long period of consistent relationship, as well as appropriate diagnostic evaluation. Such programs, however, offer a unique educational opportunity for geriatricians to learn to evaluate and treat the emotional illness in relation to medical and neurological treatment.

At Boston University a home psychiatric service has been established (SOMA Geriatric Program/AoA Grant No. 90-A-1614) and will be one site for the Geriatric Fellowship Program, which is training physicians in the Departments of Psychiatry, Medicine, and Neurology (AoA Grant No. 90-AT-2054/01). This program has been successful over the past few years in maintaining at home many multiproblem elderly patients who have been in severe danger of institutionalization.

Index

Acute care, 77, 78, 99
   costs of, 24
   emphasis on, 35–39, 85, 103, 104
   geriatrics teaching in facilities for,
      35–39, 86
   geriatrics units in facilities for, 9,
      35–39, 92, 217
   long-term care compared to, 42, 43,
      46
   and team approach/consultative ser-
      vice, 37–39, 221
   University of Rochester (MCH)
      facilities for, 45–46
   See also crisis intervention; ill-
      ness(es); site of care
Administration on Aging (AoA), 58,
      183–184
   SOMA Geriatric Program, 229
Adult continuing education. *See* con-
      tinuing medical attention
After care, 19, 39. *See also* rehabilita-
      tion
Aging and Medical Education (National
      Academy of Sciences report), 5,
      88, 183, 191
AHEC. *See* Area Health Education
      Center(s)
Aluminum levels, 156
Alveolar macrophages, 166, 168. *See
      also* pneumonia, bacterial
Alzheimer disease (AD). *See* senile
      dementia
Ambulatory care, 19, 22, 77, 191
   national perspective on, 103–107
   and office visits, 104–107, 185
   as phase of geriatric life, 60, 61, 63,
      64
   transportation as problem in, 105,
      186, VA, 49, 51, 55
   See also day care, adult; home care
American Association of Retired Per-
      sons (AARP), 72, 189

NRTA-AARP Andrus Foundation,
      73
American Geriatrics Society, 4, 189
   curriculum development contract
      awarded to, 87
   education recommendations by,
      190–191
   Journal of, 187, 189
Anderson, W.F., 17
Andrus, Ethel Percy, and Andrus
      Foundation, 73–74
Area Agencies on Aging, 19, 22, 58,
      62. *See also* community-service
      agencies
Area Health Education Bill, 201. *See
      also* legislation
Area Health Education Center(s)
      (AHEC): University of Mary-
      land, 184, 201–207. *See also*
      team-care approach
Arthritis, 74. *See also* illness(es)
Ashwroth, H.W., 99
Aspiration, "silent." *See* pneumonia,
      bacterial
Assessment. *See* evaluation and place-
      ment
Assessment and Placement Service
      (APS, Canada), 31
Association of Professors of Medicine,
      6
Atherosclerosis, 144, 149. *See also* car-
      diovascular system; senile de-
      mentia
Attitudes toward elderly, 112–113
   negative, 8, 10, 86, 93–94, 113,
      114, 187, 188, 221
   positive, development of, 62, 86,
      88, 94, 107, 189, 190
   site of care as factor in, 213
   See also doctor-patient relationship

Ball, M.J., 153